COMPREHENSIVE DIABETES CARE

Dr. Barry R. Putney

Copyright © 2024 by Dr. Barry R. Putney

All rights reserved. No part of this publication may be reproduced, distributed, or transmitted in any form or by any means, including photocopying, recording, or other electronic or mechanical methods, without the prior written permission of the publisher, except in the case of brief quotations embodied in critical reviews and certain other noncommercial uses permitted by copyright law.

Foreword

Diabetes is a constantly evolving condition. Scientific advancements are accelerating, enhancing our understanding, yet substantial gaps remain, particularly regarding the mechanisms behind type 2 diabetes. Keeping pace with these developments is increasingly challenging, though numerous resources are available. Many individuals rely on the internet, utilizing both specialized websites and general search engines. However, a significant number of people still prefer printed materials, valuing a comprehensive and accessible collection of information. This volume meets that need, offering a series of up-to-date, well-referenced, scholarly articles that cover various aspects of diabetes and its underlying science. It is remarkably thorough, addressing all facets of the pathophysiology, treatment, and care of diabetes patients.

The book opens with an engaging historical essay, a must-read for anyone who picks it up. This essay reminds us of the forgotten valuable information and the lessons learned from the pre-internet era. It discusses the potential use of HbA1c for diabetes diagnosis, reflecting a significant shift from the traditional reliance on glucose measurement, a method in use for over a century. The global diabetes pandemic is examined, noting that few populations are unaffected. Each type of diabetes is described, along with their known pathophysiology. Essays on non-classical type 1 and type 2 diabetes are particularly insightful.

Comprehensive coverage is given to diabetes management and treatment, from education and lifestyle modification to the use of oral agents and insulin. The book includes valuable chapters on the often-overlooked psychological and social aspects of the disease and discusses different models of care. Complications are addressed extensively, with the book providing valuable information on less well-defined issues in diabetes patients.

The final section looks towards the future, exploring new drugs for type 1 and type 2 diabetes, as well as the potential for stem cell therapy, islet cell transplantation, and gene therapy. These discussions are both thought-provoking and informative.

Overall, this volume is an essential resource for anyone interested in diabetes. It should be available in every setting where diabetes care is provided, serving as an excellent reference guide.

Barry R. Putney
Advocacy Researcher,
Diabetes UK.

Abbreviations List

AA - Arachidonic Acid
AAA - Abdominal Aortic Aneurysm
AACE - American Association of Clinical Endocrinologists
AADE - American Association of Diabetes Educators
ABI - Ankle Brachial Index
ACA - Acetyl Coenzyme A
ACC - Acetyl-CoA Carboxylase
ACEi - Angiotensin-Converting Enzyme Inhibitor
ACR - Albumin:Creatinine Ratio
ACS - Acute Coronary Syndromes
ACTH - Adrenocorticotropic Hormone
ADA - American Diabetes Association
ADASP - Autoimmune Diabetes in Adults with Slowly Progressive β-Cell Failure
ADI - Acceptable Daily Intake
AGE - Advanced Glycation End-Product
AGRP - Agouti-Related Peptide
ALT - Alanine Aminotransferase

AMI- Acute Myocardial Infarction
AMPK - Adenosine Monophosphate-Activated Protein Kinase
APC - Antigen-Presenting Cell
ARB - Angiotensin Receptor Blocker
AST - Aspartate Aminotransferase
AT - Angiotensin
ATG - Antithymocyte Globulin
BB - Bio-Breeding
BCG- Bacille Calmette-Guérin
BIPSS- Bilateral Inferior Petrosal Sinus Sampling
BMD - Bone Mineral Density
BMI - Body Mass Index
BNP - B-Type Natriuretic Peptide
BP - Blood Pressure
BUN - Blood Urea Nitrogen
CABG - Coronary Artery Bypass Grafting
CAD - Coronary Artery Disease
CaMK- Calcium/Calmodulin-Dependent Kinase
cAMP - Cyclic Adenosine Monophosphate
CA-MRSA - Community-Associated Methicillin-Resistant Staphylococcus Aureus
CAP - Cbl Associated Protein

CAPD - Continuous Ambulatory Peritoneal Dialysis
CART - Cocaine and Amphetamine-Related Transcript
CBF - Cerebral Blood Flow
CBT - Cognitive-Behavioral Therapy
CCA - Calcium-Channel Antagonist
CCK - Cholecystokinin
CCM - Chronic Care Model
CD - Celiac Disease
CDC - Centers for Disease Control and Prevention
CDFC - Comprehensive Diabetic Foot Examination
CDK - Cyclin-Dependent Kinase
CEL - Carboxyl Ester Lipase
CETP - Cholesterol Ester Transfer Protein
CFTR - Cystic Fibrosis Transmembrane Conductance Regulator
CGM - Continuous Glucose Monitoring
CGMP - Cyclic Guanosine Monophosphate
CGMS - Continuous Glucose Monitoring Systems
CGRP - Calcitonin Gene-Related Peptide

CHD - Coronary Heart Disease
CHF - Congestive Heart Failure
CHO - Chinese Hamster Ovary
CI - Confidence Interval
cIMT - Carotid Intima-Media Thickness
CKD - Chronic Kidney Disease
CML - Carboxymethyl Lysine
CN - Charcot Neuroarthropathy
CNV - Copy Number Variant
CoA - Coenzyme A
COX - Cyclo-Oxygenase
CPLA2 - Cytosolic Phospholipase A2
CPT - Carnitine Palmitoyltransferase
CRH - Corticotropin-Releasing Hormone
CRP - C-Reactive Protein
CRS - Congenital Rubella Syndrome
CSII - Continuous Subcutaneous Insulin Infusion
CsA - Cyclosporine A
CT - Computed Tomography
CTGF - Connective Tissue Growth Factor
CVD - Cardiovascular Disease
DAG - Diacylglycerol

DASP - Diabetes Antibody Standardization Program
DAWN - Diabetes Attitudes, Wishes, and Needs Study
DCCT - Diabetes Control and Complications Trial
DD - Disc Diameter
DEXA - Dual-Energy X-ray Absorptiometry
DHA - Docosahexaenoic Acid
DHEA - Dehydroepiandrosterone
DIDMOAD - Diabetes Insipidus, Diabetes Mellitus, Optic Atrophy, and Deafness
DISH - Diffuse Idiopathic Skeletal Hyperostosis
DKA - Diabetic Ketoacidosis
DM - Diabetic Maculopathy
DPN - Distal Symmetrical Sensory or Sensorimotor Polyneuropathy
DPP - Diabetes Prevention Program
DPP-4 - Dipeptidyl Peptidase 4
DQOL - Diabetes Quality of Life
DR - Diabetic Retinopathy
DRS - Diabetic Retinopathy Study
DSA - Digital Subtraction Angiography
DSME - Diabetes Self-Management Education

DVLA - Driver and Vehicle Licensing Agency
DVT - Deep Venous Thrombosis
DZ - Dizygotic
EAG - Estimated Average Glucose Measurement
ECG - Electrocardiography/Electrocardiogram
ED - Erectile Dysfunction
EDHF - Endothelium-Derived Hyperpolarizing Factor
EDIC - Epidemiology of Diabetes Interventions and Complications
EDNOS - Eating Disorder Not Otherwise Specified
EEG - Electroencephalography/Electroencephalogram
EGFR - Estimated Glomerular Filtration Rate
ELISA - Enzyme-Linked Immunosorbent Assay
ELISPOT - Enzyme-Linked Immunospot Assay
EMEA - European Medicines Agency
ENOS - Endothelial Nitric Oxide Synthase
EPA - Eicosapentaenoic Acid
EPC - Endothelial Progenitor Cell
ER - Endoplasmic Reticulum
ERCP - Endoscopic Retrograde Cholangiopancreatography

ERK - Extracellular Signal-Regulated Kinase
ERM - Ezrin-Radixin-Moesin
ESCS - Electrical Spinal Cord Stimulation
ESRD - End-Stage Renal Disease
ESRF - End-Stage Renal Failure
ET - Endothelin
ETDRS - Early Treatment Diabetic Retinopathy Study
EVAR - Endovascular Aneurysm Repair
FADH2 - Flavin Adenine Dinucleotide
FAS - Fatty Acid Synthase
FCPD - Fibrocalculous Pancreatic Diabetes
FDA - Food and Drug Administration
FDG - [18F]-2-Deoxy-2-Fluoro-D-Glucose
FDGF - Fibroblast-Derived Growth Factor
FDR - First-Degree Relative
FFA - Free Fatty Acid
FHWA - Federal Highways Administration
FPD - Fibrous Proliferation at the Disc
FPE - Fibrous Proliferation Elsewhere
FPG - Fasting Plasma Glucose
FPIR - First-Phase Insulin Release
FSGS - Focal Segmental Glomerulosclerosis
FSH - Follicle Stimulating Hormone

GABA - γ-Aminobutyric Acid
GAD - Glutamine Acid Decarboxylase
GAG - Glycosaminoglycan
GAPDH - Glyceraldehyde-3-Phosphate Dehydrogenase
GAS - Group A Streptococcus
GDM - Gestational Diabetes Mellitus
GFA - Glutamine:Fructose-6-Amidotransferase
GFR- Glomerular Filtration Rate
GH - Growth Hormone
GHb - Glycated Hemoglobin
GHBP - Growth Hormone-Binding Protein
GHD - Growth Hormone Deficiency
GHRH - Growth Hormone-Releasing Hormone
GI - Glycemic Index
GIP - Glucose-Dependent Insulinotropic Peptide

Preface
Abbreviations

CONTENTS

CHAPTER ONE: THE HISTORY OF DIABETES MELLITUS

- Early Discoveries and Theories
  - Discovery by Minkowski and von Mering (1889)
    - Debate on Pancreas Function
    - Concept of Internal Secretions
- Understanding Diabetes Complexity
  - Heterogeneity of Diabetes
  - Contributions of Claude Bernard
- Clinical Observations in the 19th Century
  - Identification of Diabetic Retinopathy by Jaeger (1869)
  - Nerve Damage Observations by Rollo and de Calvi
  - Kidney Disease in Diabetes by Griesinger
- Emergence of Different Diabetes Types

- Classification by Lancereaux (1880)
- The 20th Century and Insulin Discovery
  - Early Attempts to Cure Diabetes
  - Insulin Isolation by Banting and Best (1921)
  - First Clinical Trial of Insulin (1922)
- Post-Insulin Era
  - Transformation of Diabetes Management
  - Challenges: Hypoglycemia and Chronic Kidney Disease

CHAPTER TWO: CLASSIFICATION AND DIAGNOSIS OF DIABETES MELLITUS

- Introduction
  - Overview of Diabetes Mellitus
  - Importance of Classification and Diagnosis
- Definitions and Classification
  - Type 1 Diabetes (T1DM): Autoimmune Destruction of Beta Cells
  - Type 2 Diabetes (T2DM): Insulin Resistance and Relative Insulin Deficiency
  - Other Specific Types: Genetic Defects, Pancreatic Diseases, Endocrinopathies, Drug-Induced Diabetes

- Gestational Diabetes Mellitus (GDM): Hyperglycemia During Pregnancy, Risks to Mother and Fetus
- Intermediate Hyperglycemia
  - Impaired Glucose Tolerance (IGT)
  - Impaired Fasting Glucose (IFG)
  - High-Risk States for Future Diabetes and Cardiovascular Disease
- Diagnosis Methods
  - HbA1c Testing: Measurement of Average Blood Sugar Levels, Advantages
  - Glucose Measurement and Monitoring: Self-Monitoring Devices
- Trends in Incidence Over Time
  - Global Trends in T1DM Incidence: Late 20th Century Increase, Regional Variations
- Familial Clustering and Twin Studies
  - Genetic Influence on T1DM: Increased Risk in First-Degree Relatives, Concordance Rates
  - Role of Environmental Factors: Viral Infections, Hygiene Hypothesis, Dietary Factors

CHAPTER THREE: EPIDEMIOLOGY OF TYPE 2 DIABETES MELLITUS (T2DM)

- Introduction
  - Global Prevalence of T2DM
  - Ethnic and Regional Variations
  - Projections and Contributing Factors
- Diagnostic Criteria and Epidemiological Implications
  - Evolution of Diagnostic Thresholds
  - Impact of IFG and IGT
  - Changes in Dysglycemia Categorization
- Risk Factors
  - Age and Obesity: Impact of Advancing Age, Central Obesity and T2DM Risk

CHAPTER FOUR: ISLET FUNCTION AND INSULIN SECRETION

- Overview
  - Importance of Islet Function
  - Role of β-cells in Metabolic Homeostasis
- Insulin Secretion Mechanisms
  - Integration of Nutrient Sensing and Cellular Signaling
  - Neural and Hormonal Inputs

- Glucose Sensing and ATP Production
  - Glucose Transport and Metabolism
- Role of Calcium in Insulin Exocytosis
  - Insulin Granule Exocytosis
- Storage and Release of Insulin
  - Granule Dynamics: Cytoplasmic and Plasma Membrane Pools
- Regulation of Insulin Secretion
  - Nutrient-Induced Secretion
  - Neural and Hormonal Modulation
- Cellular Signaling Pathways
  - KATP Channel-Dependent Initiation
  - Calcium Signaling and Exocytosis
- Clinical Implications and Therapeutic Strategies
  - Insights into Diabetes Therapies
  - Therapeutic Approaches
- Future Directions in Research
  - Genetic Studies: Genome-Wide Association Studies
  - Emerging Technologies: Live-Cell Imaging, Pharmacological Interventions

CHAPTER FIVE: INSULIN SIGNALING PATHWAYS AND BIOLOGICAL EFFECTS

- Insulin Receptor and Intracellular Signal Transduction
  - Structural and Functional Insights
  - Regulation and Dysfunction
- Insulin Signaling Pathways and Negative Modulatory Effects
  - Role of PI3 Kinase
  - Activation of PI3 Kinase
- Insulin Receptor Substrate Proteins (IRS)
  - Signal Transduction Mechanism
  - Tyrosine Phosphorylation and SH2 Domain Protein Recruitment
  - Enzymatic Activities Propagating Insulin Signals
  - Pathogenic Roles in Insulin Resistance
  - Tissue-Specific Roles of IRS1 and IRS2
- Inhibition of Insulin Signal Transduction
  - Mechanisms of Inhibition
  - Impact on Metabolic Responses
  - Contribution to Insulin Resistance

CHAPTER SIX: DOMAIN STRUCTURE AND FUNCTION IN BIOLOGY

- Types of Domains
  - Significance of Domains
  - Functional Specificity
- Evolutionary Insights
  - Structural Features: Folded Architecture, Domain Interactions
- Biomedical Implications
  - Disease Mechanisms
  - Drug Development
- Maturity-Onset Diabetes of the Young (MODY)
  - Types of MODY and Associated Genes
  - Genetic and Clinical Diversity
  - Diagnosis and Management

CHAPTER SEVEN: INSULIN SECRETION DYNAMICS AND β-CELL FUNCTION IN TYPE 2 DIABETES

- Importance of Insulin Secretion Dynamics
  - Appropriateness of Plasma Insulin Levels

- Role of β-Cell Defects in T2DM Progression
- Insulin Secretion Abnormalities in T2DM
- Genetic and Acquired Factors Influencing β-Cell Function
- Histological Features of Islets in T2DM

CHAPTER EIGHT: INSULIN RESISTANCE IN TYPE 2 DIABETES

- Insulin Resistance in Tissues
- Chronic Hyperglycemia and Insulin Sensitivity
- Definitions and Role of Insulin
- Insulin Resistance and Its Broader Effects
- Debate: Insulin Resistance vs. β-Cell Failure

CHAPTER NINE: DRUG-INDUCED DIABETES

- Insulin Resistance in the Liver
- Acquired Causes of Hepatic Insulin Sensitivity Variation
- Insulin Resistance in Adipose Tissue

CHAPTER TEN: METABOLIC DISTURBANCES IN DIABETES

- Hyperglycemia
  - Defining Metabolic Abnormality in Diabetes
  - Variations in Underlying Abnormalities Across Diabetes Subgroups
- Carbohydrate Metabolism
  - Fasting State
  - Postprandial State
  - Insulin Secretion Response to Glucose Levels
  - Splanchnic and Muscle Glucose Disposal
- Insulin Resistance in Diabetes
  - Variations in Insulin Resistance in T1DM and T2DM
  - Role of Insulin in Glucose Uptake and Suppression of Endogenous Glucose Production
- Insulin and Glucose Regulation in Lipid Metabolism
  - Adipose Tissue and Muscle LPL Activity
  - Insulin and Glucose Roles in Lipid Metabolism

- Delayed LPL Activation and Increased FFA Levels in T2DM
- Protein Metabolism in Diabetes
  - Insulin's Role in Protein Synthesis and Breakdown
  - Urinary Nitrogen Excretion and Insulin Therapy Effects
- Lipid Metabolism in Diabetes
  - Triglyceride Dynamics
  - Energy Storage and Mobilization of Triglycerides
  - FFA Uptake and Re-esterification Processes
- Hormonal Regulation of Lipolysis
  - Hormone-Sensitive Lipase and Insulin Regulation
  - Insulin Deficiency and Its Effects on FFA Levels
- Insulin Deficiency and FFA Dynamics
  - Impact of Insulin Deficiency in T1DM
  - Insulin Counteraction of Other Hormone Effects
- Exercise and FFA Availability
  - Effects of Moderate-Intensity Exercise on FFA and Insulin Levels

- Ketoacidosis and Its Triggers
  - Physical Stress and Hormonal Responses
  - Triggers of Ketoacidosis and Hormonal Influences
  - Osmotic Diuresis and Electrolyte Imbalance
- Acidosis and Cardiovascular Implications
  - Role of Ketone Bodies and Glucose in Osmotic Diuresis
  - Metabolic Acidosis Effects and Potential Outcomes

CHAPTER ELEVEN: OBESITY AND DIABETES

- Introduction
  - Global Epidemic
  - Health Implications
  - Relationship with Diabetes
- Definition and Body Fat Distribution
  - BMI Classification by WHO
  - Prevalence of Overweight and Obesity
  - Importance of Waist Circumference
- Obesity as a Risk Factor for T2DM
  - Clinical Data on Body Fat and Diabetes Risk

- Impact of Weight Gain on Diabetes Risk
- Genetic Factors and Obesity
  - Genetic Influences

CHAPTER TWELVE: MONOGENIC CAUSES OF DIABETES

Monogenic Diabetes Types
- Glucokinase MODY
- Pathophysiology
- Clinical Features
- Differentiation from Type 1 and Type 2 Diabetes
- Management
- Pregnancy Considerations
- Transcription Factor MODY

Common Mutations (HNF1A, HNF4A)
- Clinical Features
- Differentiation from Type 1 and Type 2 Diabetes
- Management
- Pregnancy Considerations

Neonatal Diabetes
- Overview and Prevalence
- Genetic Causes
- Clinical Features
- Management
- Genetic Counseling

CHAPTER THIRTEEN: ENDOCRINE DISORDERS CAUSING DIABETES

Acromegaly
- Overview
- Features of Glucose Intolerance in Acromegaly

Cushing Syndrome
- Management of Cushing Syndrome

Pheochromocytomas: Causes and Symptoms
- Case Presentation: Emergency Management of Pheochromocytoma
- Diagnosis and Management of Pheochromocytoma
- Outcome of Pheochromocytoma and Glucose Tolerance

- Mechanisms of Hyperglycemia in Pheochromocytoma

Other Endocrine Conditions Affecting Glucose Tolerance
- Glucagonoma
- Somatostatinoma
- VIPoma

CHAPTER FOURTEEN: PANCREATIC DISEASES AND DIABETES

Introduction
- Overview of pancreatic diseases

Acute Pancreatitis
- Symptoms and causes of acute pancreatitis
- Metabolic abnormalities and transient hyperglycemia
- Potential for permanent diabetes in severe cases

Chronic Pancreatitis
- Irreversible exocrine tissue

- Regional causes

Tropical Calcific Pancreatitis
- Characteristics and prevalence
- Association with pancreatic calcification

Hereditary Hemochromatosis
- Iron deposition in pancreatic islets leading to diabetes
- Secondary hemochromatosis in conditions

CHAPTER FIFTEEN: CLINICAL PRESENTATION OF DIABETES

Clinical Considerations at Presentation
- Understanding patient perspectives and beliefs about diabetes
- Differentiating between types of diabetes based on clinical history and symptoms

Types of Diabetes
- Overview of diabetes classification: T1DM, T2DM, monogenic diabetes, and secondary forms

- Tailored management strategies for each subtype

Management Implications
- Indications for insulin therapy based on clinical presentation
- Early intervention to mitigate diabetes-related risks

Clinical Features of Diabetes Presentation
- Thirst and Urinary Symptoms
- Renal Threshold and Glycosuria
- Age-Related Considerations
- Weight Loss
- Infections
- Blurred Vision
- Rare Infections

Diabetic Ketoacidosis (DKA)
- Pathophysiology and clinical manifestations
- Diagnostic criteria and urgent management strategies

Hyperosmolar Hyperglycemic Syndrome (HSS)

- Characteristics specific to T2DM patients
- Clinical presentation and management approaches

Macrovascular Presentations
- Acute Myocardial Infarction (AMI)
- Acute Stroke

Microvascular Presentations
- Eye Presentations
- Foot Lesions

Pregnancy
- Gestational diabetes mellitus (GDM)
- Risk factors and screening recommendations

CHAPTER SIXTEEN: THE AIMS OF DIABETES CARE

Introduction
- Overview of diabetes as a chronic condition with significant health implications
- Importance of effective management in reducing mortality and morbidity risks

St. Vincent's Declaration
- Historical perspective on the shift towards patient-centered diabetes care
- Emphasis on patient responsibility and collaborative care for enhanced management outcomes

The Diabetes Care Team
- Multidisciplinary approach to diabetes care involving various healthcare professionals
- Importance of continuity and personalized care in managing diabetes

Improving Consultation Outcomes
- Strategies for optimizing patient-provider interactions during diabetes consultations
- Importance of preparation, effective communication, and shared decision-making

Interactions Between Diabetes Patients and Healthcare Professionals
- Promoting mutual understanding and active patient participation in care

- Strategies for fostering collaborative management and ongoing support

Following Diagnosis
- Critical period post-diagnosis requiring support and education
- Importance of tailored medical examinations and personalized care plans

Diabetes Education
- Role of ongoing education in equipping patients with necessary self-management skills
- Adaptation of educational initiatives to reflect current medical advancements

Glycemic Targets and Lipid Profile Recommendations
- Comparison of glycated hemoglobin (HbA1c) and lipid profile targets by authoritative bodies

Optimal Glycemic Control and Complications
- Findings from Diabetes Control and Complications Trial (DCCT) and UK Prospective Diabetes Study (UKPDS)

- Challenges and strategies in achieving optimal glycemic control

Hypoglycemia Management
- Impact of hypoglycemia on diabetes management
- Strategies for prevention, recognition, and treatment of hypoglycemic episodes

Personalized Glycemic Targets
- Considerations for setting individualized glycemic goals
- Balancing strict glycemic control with risk of hypoglycemia and other complications

Nuanced Approach to Glycemic Control
- Insights from clinical trials on intensive glycemic control and cardiovascular outcomes
- Importance of personalized treatment approaches based on individual health profiles

CHAPTER ONE

THE HISTORY OF DIABETICS MELLITUS

Early Discoveries and Theories

In 1889, Oskar Minkowski and Josef von Mering made a pivotal discovery while investigating fat metabolism. They found that removing a dog's pancreas induced severe diabetes. This accidental finding underscored the pancreas's role in regulating blood sugar levels. Minkowski noted the dog's excessive urination (polyuria) and subsequently tested its urine for sugar.

During this time, there was debate over whether the pancreas removed a diabetogenic toxin or produced an internal secretion controlling carbohydrate metabolism. The concept of "internal secretions" gained traction after

Charles-Édouard Brown-Séquard's 1889 rejuvenation claims from testicular extract injections. This idea was further supported in 1891 when sheep thyroid extract was reported to treat myxedema.

In 1893, Gustave Laguesse proposed that the pancreas's internal secretion originated from the "islets" of cells within its tissue, initially identified by Paul Langerhans in 1869. Laguesse coined the term "islets of Langerhans," and in 1909, Jean de Meyer suggested the name "insulin" for their hypothetical glucose-lowering secretion.

Understanding Diabetes Complexity

Minkowski's findings did not immediately clarify diabetes's origins. Over the subsequent two decades, diabetes was recognized as a heterogeneous disorder involving multiple organs such as the brain, pancreas, and liver. Claude Bernard's 19th-century discovery of liver glycogen and his findings linking nervous system lesions to temporary hyperglycemia suggested nervous influences on diabetes.

Clinical Observations in the 19th Century

During the 19th century, physicians described various diabetes complications. Eduard von Jaeger first identified diabetic retinopathy in 1869, with Julius Hirschberg detailing its specific characteristics by 1890. Meanwhile, nerve damage in diabetic patients was noted by Rollo in the 18th century and later by Charles Marchal de Calvi in 1864. Kidney disease in diabetes was also recognized, with Wilhelm Griesinger reporting renal changes in autopsied diabetic patients in 1859.

Emergence of Different Diabetes Types

By the late 19th century, it became evident that diabetes existed in distinct forms. Etienne Lancereaux classified patients into lean (diabète maigre) and obese (diabète gras) categories in

1880, laying the groundwork for future etiological classifications.

The 20th Century and Insulin Discovery

In the early 20th century, attempts to cure diabetes with pancreatic extracts, inspired by successful treatments for myxedema, were largely unsuccessful until 1921. Frederick Banting, influenced by Moses Barron's article, hypothesized that the pancreatic principle was digested by trypsin and devised a method to extract it without degradation. Banting, along with Charles Best, successfully isolated insulin from the pancreas, with significant contributions from biochemist James Collip.

The first clinical trial of insulin in 1922 on Leonard Thompson marked a breakthrough, significantly reducing blood sugar levels and eliminating glycosuria and ketonuria. Insulin's discovery rapidly gained global recognition, leading to Banting and Macleod receiving the Nobel Prize in 1923.

Post-Insulin Era

Insulin transformed diabetes from an acute, often fatal disease to a chronic condition with long-term complications. While it saved many lives, it also introduced challenges such as hypoglycemia and chronic kidney disease. Strategies to prevent these complications continue to be critical in diabetes management.

Conclusion

The recognition that diabetes is not a single disease has driven research into its causes and treatments. The distinction between type 1 and type 2 diabetes originated from early observations and was further refined by research into insulin sensitivity and resistance. Ongoing research remains vital in understanding and managing diabetes effectively.

CHAPTER TWO

CLASSIFICATION AND DIAGNOSIS OF DIABETES MELLITUS

Introduction

Persistent hyperglycemia, which can be caused by abnormalities in insulin secretion, action, or both, is a hallmark of diabetes mellitus, a chronic metabolic illness. The classification and diagnosis of diabetes have evolved significantly, driven by advances in understanding its pathophysiology and clinical presentation.

Definitions and Classification

Diabetes mellitus is classified into several types:

1. Type 1 Diabetes (T1DM): Characterized by autoimmune destruction of pancreatic beta cells, leading to absolute insulin deficiency.
2. Type 2 Diabetes (T2DM): Results from insulin resistance combined with relative insulin deficiency.
3. Other Specific Types: Includes genetic defects in beta cell function, pancreatic diseases, endocrinopathies, and drug or chemical-induced diabetes.
4. Gestational Diabetes Mellitus (GDM): Hyperglycemia first detected during pregnancy, with risks to both mother and fetus.

Intermediate Hyperglycemia

Intermediate hyperglycemia includes impaired glucose tolerance (IGT) and impaired fasting glucose (IFG). These conditions indicate high-risk states for future diabetes and cardiovascular disease.

HbA1c Testing: This test measures average blood sugar levels over a recent period and is frequently utilized for diagnosis because of its ease and reliability.

Glucose Measurement and Monitoring

Accurate glucose measurement is critical for diagnosis and ongoing management of diabetes. Advances in technology have improved the reliability and convenience of glucose monitoring methods, including self-monitoring devices and continuous glucose monitors (CGMs).

Trends in Incidence Over Time

Global trends in T1DM incidence show a significant increase:

1. Late 20th Century: Marked rise in incidence rates globally, particularly in younger age groups.

2. Regional Variations: Higher rates in North America and Europe compared to Central America and Asia during the 1990s.

These trends suggest a complex interplay of genetic predisposition and environmental triggers driving the increase in T1DM cases.

Familial Clustering and Twin Studies

Genetic factors significantly influence T1DM:

1. First-Degree Relatives: Increased risk compared to the general population.
2. Monozygotic Twins: Higher concordance rates compared to dizygotic twins, indicating genetic susceptibility.

However, the fact that not all genetically susceptible individuals develop T1DM highlights the role of environmental factors in disease progression.

Environmental and Nutritional Factors

Various environmental factors may contribute to T1DM development:

1. Viral Infections: Linked to increased risk, particularly enteroviruses.
2. Hygiene Hypothesis: Reduced microbial exposure may increase autoimmune diseases.
3. Dietary Factors: Cow's milk, vitamin D, and n-3 fatty acids implicated; evidence for protective effects is mixed.

Understanding these factors is crucial for developing preventive strategies against T1DM.

Perinatal Factors and Postnatal Growth

Factors during pregnancy and early life influence T1DM risk:

1. Maternal Age and Birth Weight: Older maternal age and higher birth weight associated with increased risk.
2. Postnatal Growth: Faster growth patterns linked to higher T1DM risk, influenced by genetic predisposition.

Conclusion

T1DM is a complex disease influenced by genetic predisposition and environmental factors. While genetic susceptibility plays a critical role, environmental triggers such as viral infections and dietary factors also contribute to disease onset. Understanding these interactions is essential for developing targeted preventive measures and improving outcomes for individuals at risk of T1DM. Ongoing research continues to unravel the complexities of T1DM pathogenesis and identify opportunities for primary prevention and intervention strategies.

CHAPTER THREE
EPIDEMIOLOGY OF TYPE 2 DIABETES MELLITUS (T2DM)

Introduction

Type 2 diabetes mellitus (T2DM) is a widespread chronic disease affecting diverse ethnic groups globally. It constitutes approximately 85% of diabetes cases in Caucasians and nearly all cases in certain non-Caucasian populations. As of 2010, an estimated 285 million people worldwide had diabetes, with significant prevalence in less developed regions. The prevalence is projected to rise substantially by 2030, driven by factors such as urbanization, sedentary lifestyles, and dietary changes.

Diagnostic Criteria and Epidemiological Implications

The epidemiology of T2DM is influenced by evolving diagnostic criteria:

1. Diagnostic Thresholds: Changes in fasting glucose thresholds have impacted the identification of diabetes and prediabetic states.
2. IFG and IGT: Introduction of impaired fasting glucose (IFG) and impaired glucose tolerance (IGT) has influenced epidemiological studies by altering the categorization of dysglycemia states over time

Risk Factors

Several factors contribute to the increasing prevalence of T2DM:

1. Age and Obesity: Advancing age and obesity, particularly central obesity, are significant risk factors.

2. Lifestyle: Sedentary lifestyles, high animal fat intake, and urbanization contribute to the rising prevalence.
3. Metabolic Syndrome: Components such as hypertension and dyslipidemia further exacerbate risk.
4. Environmental Factors: Exposure to pollutants, early life events like low birth weight, and fetal malnutrition also play roles.

Emerging Risk Factors

Recent studies have identified additional risk factors:

1. Insufficient Sleep: Associated with impaired glucose tolerance and increased diabetes risk.
2. Medications: Certain medications like thiazide diuretics and antipsychotics have metabolic effects increasing diabetes risk

CHAPTER FOUR
ISLET FUNCTION AND INSULIN SECRETION

Overview

Understanding the intricate processes governing islet function and insulin secretion is essential for comprehending diabetes and metabolic disorders. Islets of Langerhans, comprising various endocrine cells, including insulin-producing β-cells, play a pivotal role in maintaining metabolic homeostasis.

Insulin Secretion Mechanisms

Insulin secretion from pancreatic β-cells is a highly regulated process crucial for maintaining glucose homeostasis. This involves intricate mechanisms integrating nutrient sensing, cellular signaling pathways, and neural and hormonal inputs.

Glucose Sensing and ATP Production

β-cells utilize specific mechanisms to sense and respond to glucose levels:

Glucose Transport and Metabolism
1. Mechanism: Glucose enters β-cells via GLUT transporters and is metabolized by glucokinase, generating ATP.
2. Effect: Elevated ATP levels lead to closure of ATP-sensitive potassium (KATP) channels.
3. Consequence: Membrane depolarization and calcium influx through voltage-gated calcium channels.

Role of Calcium in Insulin Exocytosis

Calcium plays a pivotal role in insulin secretion dynamics:

Insulin Granule Exocytosis

1. **Mechanism:** Calcium influx triggers insulin granule exocytosis by interacting with synaptotagmins and the SNARE complex.
2. **Process:** Facilitates fusion of insulin-containing granules with the plasma membrane.

Storage and Release of Insulin

Insulin is stored in dense-core secretory granules within β-cells:

Granule Dynamics
1. **Distribution:** Insulin granules are distributed throughout the cytoplasm, with a pool of readily-releasable granules near the plasma membrane.
2. **Facilitation:** Microtubules and microfilaments guide granule movement and facilitate docking and fusion at the plasma membrane.

Regulation of Insulin Secretion

Insulin secretion is regulated by multiple factors:

1. Nutrient-Induced Secretion
    - Glucose: Primary initiator of insulin secretion by stimulating ATP production.
    - Amino Acids: Synergize with glucose to enhance insulin release.
    - Fatty Acids: Modulate β-cell function and insulin secretion.

2. Neural and Hormonal Modulation
    - Autonomic Nervous System: Parasympathetic and sympathetic inputs regulate insulin secretion.
    - Hormones: GLP-1, GIP, and adrenaline potentiate insulin release, while somatostatin and NPY inhibit it.

Cellular Signaling Pathways

Insulin secretion involves complex signaling pathways:

Pathways Involved
1. KATP Channel-Dependent: Initiation of insulin release through ATP-sensitive KATP channel closure.
2. Calcium Signaling: Mediates exocytosis via voltage-gated channels and calcium-sensitive proteins like synaptotagmins.

Clinical Implications and Therapeutic Strategies

Insights into insulin secretion mechanisms inform diabetes therapies:

Therapeutic Approaches
1. Sulfonylureas: Target KATP channels to enhance insulin secretion.
2. Incretin-Based Therapies: GLP-1 agonists and DPP-4 inhibitors enhance insulin release and improve glycemic control.

Future Directions in Research

Advancements in research methodologies and technologies:

1. Genetic Studies: Genome-wide association studies identify genetic variants influencing β-cell function.
2. Emerging Technologies: Live-cell imaging and pharmacological interventions offer new insights into islet biology.

Conclusion

Understanding the mechanisms governing insulin secretion provides critical insights into diabetes pathophysiology and therapeutic strategies. Continued research into these mechanisms promises to uncover new therapeutic targets and improve outcomes for individuals with diabetes worldwide.

CHAPTER FIVE
INSULIN SIGNALING PATHWAYS AND BIOLOGICAL EFFECTS

Insulin Receptor and Intracellular Signal Transduction

Insulin initiates its cellular effects by binding to high-affinity insulin receptors located on the plasma membrane of target cells. These receptors are composed of α and β subunits and undergo conformational changes upon insulin binding, leading to autophosphorylation of tyrosine residues on the β-subunit. This autophosphorylation enhances the tyrosine kinase activity of the receptor, crucial for transmitting insulin signals intracellularly.

Structural and Functional Insights:
1. Insulin Receptor Composition: Heterotetrameric structure comprising α and β subunits.

2. Conformational Changes: Triggered by insulin binding, leading to enhanced tyrosine kinase activity.
3. Signaling Initiation: Autophosphorylation of tyrosine residues on the β-subunit.

Regulation and Dysfunction:
- Downregulation with Chronic Insulin Exposure: Reduced cell-surface expression observed in insulin-resistant conditions.
- Genetic Mutations and Antibodies: Cause severe insulin resistance syndromes when affecting the insulin receptor gene or blocking insulin binding.
- Structural Similarities: Shared with insulin-like growth factor 1 receptor (IGF1R), influencing growth and metabolic responses.

Insulin Signaling Pathways and Negative Modulatory Effects

Insulin signaling pathways involve intricate mechanisms that can be modulated negatively under conditions of insulin resistance, influencing metabolic and mitogenic responses.

Here is a revised version of the provided content, ensuring clarity and precision:

Role of PI3 Kinase:
- Negative Modulation: Interacts with stress-activated kinase pathways such as JNK.
- Obesity-Induced Effects: Contributes to insulin resistance associated with high-fat diets.
- Regulation of PTEN: Increases insulin resistance by degrading PIP3.

Activation of PI3 Kinase:
- Phosphorylation of Lipids: Produces PI(3,4,5)P3, essential for downstream signaling.

- Recruitment and Activation*1: Brings PH domain-containing proteins to the plasma membrane.
- PDK1-Mediated Activation: Phosphorylates Akt/PKB and atypical protein kinases (aPKCs).

Insulin Receptor Substrate Proteins (IRS)

IRS proteins are pivotal in transmitting signals downstream of activated insulin receptors, integrating metabolic and mitogenic pathways crucial for cellular responses to insulin.

Signal Transduction Mechanism:
- Tyrosine Phosphorylation: Triggered by insulin receptor activation.
- Recruitment of SH2 Domain Proteins: Enzymatic activities that propagate insulin signals.
- Pathogenic Roles: Deletion or dysfunction contributing to insulin resistance and diabetes pathogenesis.

- Tissue-Specific Roles: IRS1 in skeletal muscle; IRS2 in liver and pancreatic β-cells.

Inhibition of Insulin Signal Transduction

Insulin signaling pathways play a crucial role in regulating metabolic responses, and their inhibition underlies the development of insulin resistance, a hallmark of various metabolic disorders including diabetes mellitus.

Inhibition of the Insulin Receptor

The insulin receptor, pivotal in initiating insulin signaling cascades, is subject to negative modulation through several mechanisms:

1. Downregulation of Insulin Receptor Number
    - Mechanism: Prolonged exposure to elevated insulin levels leads to a reduction in cell surface insulin receptors.

- Consequence: Decreased insulin sensitivity due to a rightward shift in insulin dose-response curves.
- Processes: Increased receptor internalization followed by lysosomal degradation and reduced gene expression contribute to receptor loss.

2. Regulation through Serine-Threonine Phosphorylation
- Effect: Impairs insulin receptor tyrosine kinase activity.
- Involvement: Serine-threonine kinases negatively regulate insulin receptor function under conditions like insulin resistance.

3. Impact of Protein Tyrosine Phosphatases

Function: De-phosphorylated insulin receptor tyrosine residues, attenuating insulin signaling.

Examples: PTP1B and SHP2 are implicated in insulin resistance through dephosphorylation of critical insulin signaling molecules.

Plasma Differentiation Factor 1 (PC-1)

Plasma differentiation factor 1 (PC-1), also known as ectonucleotide pyrophosphatase phosphodiesterase 1, is a membrane glycoprotein with pyrophosphatase activity. PC-1 acts as an intrinsic inhibitor of insulin receptor tyrosine kinase, binding specifically to amino acids 485–599 of the insulin receptor's connecting domain. This interaction disrupts the conformational change required for autophosphorylation of the receptor's β-subunits upon insulin binding, thereby impairing insulin signaling. Elevated expression of PC-1 in muscle tissues correlates with reduced insulin sensitivity observed in conditions such as diabetes and obesity.

Ras-p38 MAPK Pathway

The Ras-p38 MAPK pathway represents a divergence from IRS-mediated signaling, focusing on cellular growth and mitogenesis:

Activation Mechanism:
- Insulin Stimulation: Insulin triggers tyrosine phosphorylation of IRS, facilitating recruitment of Grb-2/SOS complex.
- Ras Activation: Grb-2 binds SOS, activating Ras, a GTPase that initiates a kinase cascade.
- Kinase Cascade: Activated Ras recruits and activates Raf-1 kinase, which phosphorylates MEK and subsequently ERK1/2.
- Biological Effects: ERK1/2 translocates to the nucleus, where it phosphorylates transcription factors like ELK-1 and regulates gene expression related to cell growth and metabolism.

Stress-Induced Kinases

Under conditions such as nutrient excess and inflammation, stress-induced kinases like JNK and IKKβ are activated, contributing to insulin resistance:

Activation and Mechanism:
- Inflammatory Stimuli: TNF-α activates JNK and IKKβ.
- Serine Phosphorylation: These kinases phosphorylate IRS proteins, disrupting insulin signal transduction.
- Impact on Insulin Sensitivity: Increased serine phosphorylation of IRS impairs downstream insulin signaling pathways, contributing to insulin resistance [54, 55].

Protein Kinase C (PKC)

PKCs are serine-threonine kinases activated by conditions like hyperinsulinemia and hyperglycemia, contributing to insulin resistance:

Activation and Effects:

- Insulin Signaling Regulation: PKCs phosphorylate IRS proteins and the insulin receptor, disrupting their function.
- Pathophysiological Implications: Elevated PKC activity correlates with reduced insulin sensitivity observed in metabolic disorders such as diabetes.

Inhibition of Insulin Receptor Substrate Proteins

Several mechanisms regulate insulin receptor substrate proteins, affecting insulin signal transduction:

- Protein Tyrosine Phosphatases (PTPs):
- Activity and Regulation: PTP-1B and LAR dephosphorylate insulin receptor tyrosine residues, attenuating insulin signaling.
- Clinical Relevance: Increased PTP activity in tissues like skeletal muscle is associated with insulin resistance in type 2 diabetes.

Serine-Threonine Phosphorylation:
- Regulation Mechanism: Serine phosphorylation of IRS proteins inhibits their association with the insulin receptor and PI 3 kinase, impairing insulin signal transduction.
- Contribution to Insulin Resistance: Conditions promoting serine phosphorylation (e.g., high-fat diets) exacerbate insulin resistance.

Muscle Contraction: Independent Stimulation of Glucose Transport

Muscle contraction triggers GLUT-4 translocation and enhances glucose transport in muscles independently of insulin signaling pathways. This effect occurs without altering serum insulin levels or activating insulin receptors, PI 3 kinase, or Akt/PKB. The mobilization of GLUT-4 in response to exercise involves distinct intracellular pools compared to those recruited by insulin. Moreover, acute exercise and insulin exhibit partially additive effects, suggesting different mechanisms for glucose transport stimulation.

AMP-Activated Protein Kinase (AMPK):
- Activation Mechanism: Muscle contraction elevates intracellular 5′ AMP levels, activating AMPK.
- Role in Glucose Transport: AMPK activation enhances glucose uptake by modifying metabolic enzyme activities, including acetyl-CoA carboxylase (ACC), to restore ATP levels and curtail further ATP consumption.

Adipose Tissue

Adipose tissue acts as the primary site for triglyceride storage and plays crucial roles in insulin-mediated metabolic processes.

Lipogenesis:
- Insulin Stimulation: Insulin promotes lipogenesis by increasing fatty acid and

glucose availability for triglyceride synthesis.
- Key Enzymes: Activation of fatty acid synthase (FAS) and sterol regulatory element-binding protein 1 (SREBP-1) facilitates fatty acid synthesis. Insulin also enhances ATP citrate lyase activity, converting citrate to acetyl-CoA, a precursor for fatty acid synthesis.
- Lipolysis Suppression: Insulin inhibits hormone-sensitive lipase (HSL) and phosphorylation of perilipin, reducing cyclic AMP (cAMP) levels via Akt/PKB activation [68].

Liver

The liver regulates glucose metabolism through insulin-mediated pathways, impacting glycogenesis, glycogenolysis, and gluconeogenesis.

Glycogenesis/Glycogenolysis:

- Insulin Effect: Insulin promotes glycogen synthesis by activating glycogen synthase and inhibiting glycogenolysis and gluconeogenesis.
- Regulation Mechanisms: Glycogen synthase activation involves allosteric activation, membrane translocation, and inhibition via serine phosphorylation. Insulin-mediated GSK-3β inhibition further enhances glycogen accumulation.

Foxo Transcription Factors in Insulin Signaling

Foxo transcription factors modulate gene expression in response to insulin, particularly in tissues involved in glucose metabolism and cellular differentiation.

Mechanism of Action:
- Insulin Regulation: Upon insulin stimulation, Akt/PKB phosphorylates Foxo proteins (e.g., Foxo1), leading to their nuclear exclusion.

- Effects on Gene Expression: Foxo proteins regulate genes involved in gluconeogenesis (e.g., G-6-Pase, PEPCK), impacting glucose homeostasis.

Conclusion

Insulin exerts diverse effects across different tissues, regulating metabolic homeostasis through tissue-specific effector systems. Understanding these mechanisms provides insights into metabolic diseases and potential therapeutic targets. Further research into the interplay of insulin signaling pathways continues to elucidate complex regulatory networks critical for maintaining physiological glucose and lipid metabolism.

CHAPTER SIX
DOMAIN STRUCTURE AND FUNCTION IN BIOLOGY

Domains in biological contexts refer to distinct functional and/or structural units within larger macromolecules or proteins. Understanding domain architecture is crucial for elucidating molecular interactions, cellular processes, and disease mechanisms.

Types of Domains

1. Protein Domains

Definition and Characteristics: Protein domains are independently folding structural units that perform specific functions within proteins.

Examples: Catalytic domains (e.g., kinase domain), binding domains (e.g., SH2 domain), regulatory domains (e.g., DNA-binding domain).

2. DNA Domains

Functional Units: Domains within DNA sequences denote specific regions with defined functions, such as binding sites for transcription factors or regulatory elements.

Examples: Enhancer domains, promoter domains, coding domains.

Significance of Domains

1. Functional Specificity
   - Role in Protein Function: Domains confer specific biochemical activities, enabling proteins to perform precise functions like catalysis, binding, or structural support.
   - Regulation: Domain composition dictates protein regulation, including activity modulation and cellular localization.

2. Evolutionary Insights
   - Conservation and Divergence: Evolutionary conservation of domains highlights essential functions across

species, whereas domain divergence contributes to species-specific adaptations.

Structural Features

1. Folded Architecture
   - Tertiary Structure: Domains exhibit characteristic tertiary structures stabilized by intramolecular interactions (e.g., hydrophobic core, disulfide bonds).
   - Modularity: Modular organization allows domains to be combined in various arrangements to generate diverse functional proteins.

2. Domain Interactions
   - Interdomain Communication: Domains interact with each other or with ligands to orchestrate complex biological processes.
   - Allosteric Regulation: Changes in domain conformation due to ligand binding or post-translational modifications can allosterically regulate protein function.

Biomedical Implications

1. Disease Mechanisms
   - Mutational Effects: Mutations within domains can disrupt protein function, leading to diseases (e.g., cancer-causing mutations in kinase domains).
   - Therapeutic Targeting: Targeting specific domains offers opportunities for therapeutic interventions (e.g., kinase inhibitors in cancer treatment).

2. Drug Development
   - Target Validation: Identifying essential domains validates potential drug targets, guiding drug discovery efforts.
   - Structure-Based Design: Structural insights into domain interactions aid in designing novel therapeutic agents with improved specificity and efficacy.

Maturity-Onset Diabetes of the Young (MODY)

Maturity-Onset Diabetes of the Young (MODY) comprises a group of monogenic forms of diabetes characterized by early-onset, typically before the age of 25, and an autosomal dominant inheritance pattern. These forms of diabetes result from mutations in genes critical for pancreatic β-cell function.

Types of MODY and Associated Genes

1. MODY 1: HNF-4α (Hepatocyte Nuclear Factor 4 Alpha)
    - Role: HNF-4α regulates β-cell development, differentiation, and insulin secretion.
    - Clinical Features: Often presents with mild hyperglycemia that progresses slowly without insulin requirement initially.

2. MODY 2: Glucokinase
    - Function: Glucokinase plays a key role in glucose sensing and insulin release from β-cells.

- Clinical Characteristics: Typically mild hyperglycemia due to impaired glucose sensing; generally responds well to dietary management.

3. MODY 3: HNF-1α (Hepatocyte Nuclear Factor 1 Alpha)
    - Function: HNF-1α regulates gene expression in pancreatic β-cells, affecting insulin secretion.
    - Clinical Presentation: Often progressive insulin insufficiency requiring treatment; associated with renal complications in some cases.

4. MODY 4: IPF-1 (Insulin Promoter Factor 1)
    - Role: IPF-1 is involved in β-cell development and insulin gene expression.
    - Clinical Features: Variably penetrant diabetes phenotype with both mild and severe insulin deficiency observed.

5. MODY 5: HNF-1β (Hepatocyte Nuclear Factor 1 Beta)

- Function: HNF-1β regulates genes involved in pancreatic development and β-cell function.
- Clinical Characteristics: Can present with renal abnormalities in addition to diabetes; variable severity in insulin requirement.

6. MODY 6: NeuroD1 (Neurogenic Differentiation Factor 1)
    - Role: NeuroD1 is essential for pancreatic β-cell differentiation and function.
    - Clinical Presentation: Rare form with variable severity; often associated with early-onset diabetes.

Genetic and Clinical Diversity

- Ethnic Variations: Prevalence and spectrum of MODY mutations vary among populations (e.g., higher prevalence of HNF-1α mutations in certain European populations).
- Clinical Heterogeneity: MODY mutations exhibit variable penetrance and

expressivity, leading to diverse clinical presentations even within affected families.

Diagnosis and Management

- Genetic Testing: Essential for accurate diagnosis and differentiation from other forms of diabetes.
- Therapeutic Approach: Treatment strategies tailored based on the specific MODY subtype, ranging from dietary management to oral hypoglycemic agents or insulin therapy as needed.
- Long-Term Monitoring: Regular monitoring for complications, especially renal function in HNF-1α and HNF-1β MODY variants.

CHAPTER SEVEN
INSULIN SECRETION DYNAMICS AND β-CELL FUNCTION IN TYPE 2 DIABETES

Type 2 diabetes mellitus (T2DM) is a complex metabolic disorder influenced by both genetic predispositions and acquired factors that impair β-cell function and tissue insulin sensitivity. Understanding the dynamics of insulin secretion and β-cell defects is crucial for effective management and therapeutic interventions.

Importance of Insulin Secretion Dynamics

The dynamics of insulin secretion play a pivotal role in maintaining glucose homeostasis. Early studies highlighted abnormalities in insulin response patterns in individuals with impaired glucose tolerance (IGT) and T2DM, underscoring the significance of early and sustained insulin release phases.

Appropriateness of Plasma Insulin Levels

The regulation of insulin secretion is primarily governed by plasma glucose concentration. In T2DM, despite elevated 2-hour post-challenge insulin levels during oral glucose tolerance tests (OGTT), there is a notable decline in early insulin response, leading to ineffective suppression of endogenous glucose production and subsequent hyperglycemia.

Relationship between β-Cell Function and Insulin Resistance

A hyperbolic relationship exists between β-cell function and tissue insulin sensitivity. As insulin sensitivity declines due to factors such as obesity and physical inactivity, β-cells compensate by increasing insulin secretion to maintain normal glucose levels. However, this compensatory mechanism becomes inadequate over time, contributing to the progression from impaired glucose tolerance to overt T2DM.

Role of β-Cell Defects in T2DM Progression

Longitudinal studies demonstrate that β-cell dysfunction precedes the diagnosis of T2DM. Progressive deterioration in β-cell function, compounded by glucotoxicity and lipotoxicity, contributes to the gradual loss of insulin secretory capacity. This decline is evident even in individuals with impaired glucose tolerance and those genetically predisposed to diabetes.

Insulin Secretion Abnormalities in T2DM

Common abnormalities in insulin secretion observed in T2DM include reduced first-phase and diminished second-phase responses to hyperglycemia. Responses to mixed meals and non-glucose stimuli are blunted, reflecting a decline in maximal secretory capacity. Pulsatile insulin secretion patterns are disrupted, characterized by smaller and less regular secretory pulses.

Genetic and Acquired Factors Influencing β-Cell Function

T2DM is a polygenic disorder influenced by multiple genetic variants affecting β-cell function and insulin secretion pathways. Acquired factors such as hyperglycemia, increased free fatty acids, and oxidative stress further exacerbate β-cell dysfunction, leading to accelerated disease progression.

Histological Features of Islets in T2DM

Histological changes in pancreatic islets of T2DM patients include abnormal extracellular deposits of islet amyloid composed of amylin (IAPP) fibrils. These deposits, along with reduced β-cell mass and altered α-cell function, contribute to impaired insulin secretion and glucose dysregulation.

CHAPTER EIGHT
INSULIN RESISTANCE IN TYPE 2 DIABETES

Key Points

Insulin Resistance and Type 2 Diabetes Mellitus (T2DM)
- Insulin resistance precedes and predicts T2DM, often referred to as metabolic syndrome.
- Development of T2DM requires both insulin resistance and a relative defect in insulin secretion.

Metabolic Syndrome and Cardiovascular Disease
- While obesity and physical inactivity contribute to T2DM, they are less predictive of cardiovascular disease compared to a combination of metabolic syndrome risk factors.

- Diagnosis of metabolic syndrome involves measuring waist circumference, glucose, triglycerides, high-density lipoprotein (HDL) cholesterol, and blood pressure.
- Metabolic syndrome can occur in both obese and normal-weight individuals and is often associated with excess ectopic fat, particularly in the liver.

Non-Alcoholic Fatty Liver Disease (NAFLD)
- NAFLD is characterized by excess liver fat without significant alcohol consumption or other liver diseases.
- Liver fat content is closely linked to metabolic syndrome features and can predict T2DM and cardiovascular disease independently of obesity.

Insulin Resistance in Tissues

Liver
- In T2DM, liver insulin resistance impairs insulin's ability to inhibit hepatic glucose

production, causing mild hyperglycemia and increased insulin secretion.
- Insulin resistance also fails to suppress very low-density lipoprotein (VLDL) production, resulting in hypertriglyceridemia.
- Increased exchange of cholesterol esters for triglycerides decreases HDL levels, while small, dense low-density lipoprotein (LDL) particles, which are highly atherogenic, become prevalent.
- Hepatic insulin resistance correlates with liver fat content, influenced by genetic and dietary factors.

Adipose Tissue
- Insulin resistance in adipose tissue involves inflammation, reduced adiponectin production, and impaired insulin suppression of lipolysis.
- Elevated non-esterified fatty acid (NEFA) levels contribute to intrahepatic triglyceride accumulation under fasting and postprandial conditions.

- Adiponectin deficiency may also facilitate liver fat accumulation.

Skeletal Muscle
- T2DM patients exhibit reduced insulin-stimulated glucose uptake in skeletal muscle compared to non-diabetic individuals.
- Molecular defects include impaired insulin receptor substrate 1 tyrosine phosphorylation, phosphoinositide 3-kinase activation, and glucose transporter 4 translocation, which mediates insulin-stimulated glucose uptake.
- Elevated NEFA levels disrupt glucose utilization and uptake by muscle tissue.

Chronic Hyperglycemia and Insulin Sensitivity
- Chronic hyperglycemia decreases insulin sensitivity (glucose toxicity), potentially explaining the heightened insulin resistance in patients with established T2DM.

Definitions and Role of Insulin Resistance in T2DM Natural History
- Insulin resistance is defined as the inability of insulin to produce its typical biological effects at normal circulating concentrations.
- It leads to impaired suppression of endogenous glucose production and reduced peripheral glucose uptake.
- Insulin resistance also impacts VLDL cholesterol production, raising serum triglycerides, and increases NEFA flux in adipose tissue, further impairing insulin action on glucose metabolism in liver and muscle.

Insulin Resistance and Its Broader Effects

Impact on Other Functions of Insulin
- In Type 2 Diabetes Mellitus (T2DM), insulin resistance extends to its effects on

vasodilation and prevention of platelet aggregation.
- The severity of insulin resistance in T2DM can be exacerbated by various factors (detailed in Table 11.1).

Debate: Insulin Resistance vs. β-Cell Failure

Primary Defect Controversy
- There is ongoing debate about whether insulin resistance or β-cell failure is the primary defect leading to hyperglycemia in T2DM.
- Studies indicate a linear decrease in both first-phase insulin release and insulin sensitivity in individuals progressing from normal glucose tolerance to impaired glucose tolerance (IGT).
- When plasma glucose levels reach the upper limit for IGT after an oral glucose challenge, insulin levels decline and glucose levels rise, moving into the diabetic range.

- Both low insulin sensitivity and impaired first-phase insulin release are predictors of T2DM onset, implying that overt hyperglycemia development requires a relative reduction in insulin secretion (illustrated in Figure 11.1).

Pathogenesis and Significance of the Metabolic Syndrome

Definition and Clinical Features
- The metabolic syndrome is characterized by a cluster of conditions including hyperglycemia, hypertriglyceridemia, low high-density lipoprotein (HDL) cholesterol, hypertension, and central obesity.
- These conditions collectively increase cardiovascular risk significantly more than each condition individually.

International Diabetes Federation (IDF) Criteria
- According to the IDF, a diagnosis of metabolic syndrome requires central

obesity plus any two of the following: elevated triglycerides, reduced HDL cholesterol, elevated blood pressure, or elevated fasting plasma glucose.
- Approximately 20-25% of the global adult population meets these criteria, doubling their risk of cardiovascular disease and increasing their risk of developing T2DM fivefold.

Insulin Resistance in Specific Tissues

Liver
- In T2DM, liver insulin resistance results in impaired suppression of hepatic glucose production, mild hyperglycemia, and increased insulin secretion.
- Insulin resistance also leads to failure in suppressing very low-density lipoprotein (VLDL) production, resulting in hypertriglyceridemia.
- Increased cholesterol ester exchange decreases HDL levels, while small, dense low-density lipoprotein (LDL) particles

become predominant and highly atherogenic.
- The extent of hepatic insulin resistance correlates with liver fat content, which is influenced by genetic and dietary factors.

Adipose Tissue

Insulin resistance in adipose tissue involves inflammation, reduced adiponectin production, and impaired suppression of lipolysis.

Elevated non-esterified fatty acid (NEFA) levels contribute significantly to intrahepatic triglyceride accumulation.

Adiponectin deficiency may also promote liver fat accumulation.

Skeletal Muscle

Patients with T2DM exhibit decreased insulin-stimulated glucose uptake in skeletal muscle.

Molecular defects include impaired insulin receptor substrate 1 tyrosine phosphorylation,

phosphoinositide 3-kinase activation, and glucose transporter 4 translocation.
Elevated NEFA levels interfere with muscle glucose utilization and uptake.

Chronic Hyperglycemia and Insulin Sensitivity
Chronic hyperglycemia decreases insulin sensitivity, potentially worsening insulin resistance in T2DM patients.

Factors Influencing Insulin Action in T2DM

Physiological Variations
Factors such as physical training, increased muscle mass, and fat distribution can affect insulin sensitivity.

Diet-Induced Changes
Overfeeding, starvation, and the type of dietary fat can alter insulin sensitivity.

Metabolic and Electrolyte Disturbances
High free fatty acid concentrations, chronic hyperglycemia, hypoglycemia, acidosis,

hyperosmolality, and hypophosphatemia impact insulin sensitivity.

Other Contributing Factors
Conditions such as excessive secretion of counter-regulatory hormones, physical or mental stress, acromegaly, Cushing's disease, pheochromocytoma, growth hormone deficiency, thyroid disorders, non-alcoholic fatty liver, uremia, and various infections can also affect insulin sensitivity.

The Impact of Non-Alcoholic Fatty Liver Disease (NAFLD)

Metabolic Syndrome and Liver Fat Accumulation
Individuals with metabolic syndrome, especially those with abdominal obesity, often exhibit increased liver fat and hepatic insulin resistance, independent of their overall obesity and fat distribution.

This condition, known as non-alcoholic fatty liver disease (NAFLD), is characterized by excess liver fat (>5-10% histologically) not caused by alcohol consumption, toxins, autoimmune, viral, or other causes of liver steatosis.

NAFLD is a predictor of both T2DM and cardiovascular disease, irrespective of obesity.

Defining NAFLD and Its Spectrum

NAFLD encompasses a range of liver diseases, from simple steatosis to non-alcoholic steatohepatitis (NASH) and cirrhosis.

The mechanisms driving the progression from simple steatosis to NASH, characterized by liver inflammation, remain unclear.

The incidence of severe liver damage due to NAFLD is rising, paralleling the epidemics of obesity, T2DM, and cardiovascular disease.

Diagnostic Criteria for Metabolic Syndrome

International Diabetes Federation (IDF) Definition

Metabolic syndrome diagnosis requires central obesity plus any two of the following factors:

Raised triglycerides: ≥150 mg/dL (1.7 mmol/L) or treatment for this lipid abnormality.

Reduced HDL cholesterol: <40 mg/dL (1.0 mmol/L) in males and <50 mg/dL (1.3 mmol/L) in females, or treatment for this lipid abnormality.

Raised blood pressure: systolic BP ≥130 or diastolic BP ≥85 mmHg, or treatment for previously diagnosed hypertension.

Raised fasting plasma glucose: ≥100 mg/dL (5.6 mmol/L), or previously diagnosed type 2 diabetes. An oral glucose tolerance test is recommended if glucose is above 5.6 mmol/L (100 mg/dL).

For individuals with a BMI >30 kg/m^2, central obesity can be assumed without measuring waist circumference.

Ethnic-Specific Waist Circumference Values

Different ethnic groups have specific waist circumference thresholds to define central obesity.

NAFLD and Glucose Metabolism

Hepatic Insulin Resistance
In T2DM, the liver's ability to store glucose during meals is relatively intact, but the rate of glucose utilization is normal due to the mass action effect of hyperglycemia.

The primary cause of postprandial hyperglycemia is the insufficient inhibition of endogenous glucose synthesis.

Lipoprotein Metabolism
Insulin normally suppresses the production of very low-density lipoprotein (VLDL), especially VLDL apoB particles, from the liver by decreasing NEFA availability and directly inhibiting VLDL assembly.

In T2DM, insulin fails to suppress VLDL apoB production, contributing to increased serum triglycerides.

High serum triglycerides lead to reduced HDL levels and increased CETP-mediated cholesterol ester and triglyceride exchange between HDL, VLDL, and LDL particles, resulting in small, dense, and highly atherogenic LDL particles.

CHAPTER NINE
DRUG-INDUCED DIABETES

Key Points

- Many commonly used medications can disrupt glucose homeostasis, leading to hyperglycemia in non-diabetic individuals or worsening glycemic control in diabetic patients.
- Glucocorticoids can induce insulin resistance through post-insulin receptor mechanisms, often necessitating the use of oral hypoglycemic agents or insulin during treatment.
- Oral contraceptives rarely cause hyperglycemia, except in formulations with high-dose estrogen or progesterone (levonorgestrel), especially in women with a history of gestational diabetes.

- Estrogen replacement therapy in postmenopausal women does not typically affect glycemic control.
- Thiazide diuretics can impair insulin secretion, particularly at high doses, with this effect linked to potassium depletion.
- Loop diuretics like furosemide (frusemide) are less likely to cause hyperglycemia.
- Non-selective β-adrenoceptor antagonists can inhibit insulin secretion and impair glucose tolerance, whereas cardioselective β1-adrenoceptor blockers have a lesser impact.
- Other drugs that can precipitate or exacerbate hyperglycemia include:
- Streptozocin (streptozotocin), pentamidine, and ciclosporin (cyclosporine) due to β-cell toxicity.
- Diazoxide through inhibition of insulin secretion.
- β2-receptor agonists (e.g., salbutamol and ritodrine), which increase hepatic glucose production.

- Supraphysiologic doses of growth hormone.
- Protease inhibitors (e.g., indinavir, nelfinavir, ritonavir, saquinavir) by inducing insulin resistance.
- Antipsychotics through weight gain and insulin resistance.

The increasing recognition by the World Health Organization (WHO) and the American Diabetes Association (ADA) of drug-induced diabetes as a distinct etiologic category highlights the significance of this issue (see Chapter 2). Understanding the diabetogenic properties of drugs is crucial for two main reasons. First, polypharmacy is often unavoidable in diabetes management, so awareness of potential hyperglycemic effects helps in preventing and managing glycemic control deterioration. Secondly, some drugs can induce diabetes in previously normoglycemic individuals, typically a reversible and non-insulin-dependent condition but potentially permanent.

Drugs can elevate blood glucose levels through two primary mechanisms: reducing insulin production or secretion, and diminishing tissue sensitivity to insulin. Notable examples include glucocorticoids, which are widely used in various diseases.

Insulin Resistance in the Liver

Glucose Metabolism in the Fasting State
- During fasting, insulin suppresses endogenous glucose production. In T2DM, this suppression is impaired due to insulin resistance, leading to increased basal glucose production.
- Hepatic insulin resistance is linked with excess liver fat, and strategies to lower fasting glucose should focus on inhibiting hepatic glucose production rather than increasing peripheral glucose uptake.

Postprandial State
- In the postprandial state, about one-third of glucose is utilized in skeletal muscle,

one-third is oxidized in the brain, and the remaining third is stored in the liver.
- In T2DM patients, the liver's glucose storage capability remains relatively intact, but the suppression of endogenous glucose production is incomplete, contributing to postprandial hyperglycemia.

Clinical Implications
- The findings highlight the importance of targeting hepatic glucose production and lipoprotein metabolism in managing T2DM and its complications.
- Effective treatment strategies should consider the unique metabolic challenges in patients with T2DM, focusing on both fasting and postprandial glucose control.

Acquired Causes of Hepatic Insulin Sensitivity Variation

Body Weight and Distribution:

Obesity correlates with insulin resistance, but there is considerable variation in insulin sensitivity at any given BMI. Liver fat content and hepatic insulin resistance are closely related to BMI and waist circumference. Weight loss significantly reduces liver fat and improves insulin sensitivity.

.Fat Distribution:
Upper body obesity, characterized by visceral fat accumulation, is more harmful regarding insulin resistance and liver fat. Visceral fat is metabolically active and releases NEFAs into the portal vein, potentially leading to hepatic insulin resistance.

Insulin Resistance in Adipose Tissue
Adipose tissue is an active endocrine organ releasing hormones like adiponectin and leptin. In obese individuals and those with fatty liver, adipose tissue inflammation characterized by macrophage infiltration and increased pro-inflammatory molecules may cause systemic

insulin resistance, including hepatic insulin resistance.

Adiponectin Deficiency:
Adiponectin, primarily targeting the liver, has anti-inflammatory and insulin-sensitizing effects. Serum adiponectin levels are lower in obese individuals and those with metabolic syndrome, correlating with increased liver fat.

Insulin Resistance in Skeletal Muscle

Defects in the insulin signaling cascade, particularly post-receptor signaling involving IRS-1 and PI 3-kinase, reduce glucose uptake and glycogen synthesis. These defects are partially reversible with weight loss, suggesting metabolic disturbances contribute significantly to insulin resistance.

Imbalances in the Skeletal Muscle's Insulin Function

The impairments in insulin action within skeletal muscle are more severe in diabetic patients compared to equally obese, non-diabetic individuals of the same age, gender, and body fat distribution. This suggests the involvement of additional genetic defects or metabolic disturbances such as chronic hyperglycemia (glucose toxicity) or the accumulation of extracellular NEFA and lipids within myocytes (lipotoxicity).

Chronic Hyperglycemia

Hyperglycemia, independent of insulin, NEFA, or counter-regulatory hormones, can induce insulin resistance in human skeletal muscle. This phenomenon, known as "glucose toxicity," contributes to the reduced rates of insulin-stimulated glucose uptake in Type 2 Diabetes Mellitus (T2DM) patients, compared to non-diabetic subjects matched for weight, age, and gender. While chronic hyperglycemia induces insulin resistance, acute glucose utilization is still stimulated through the mass action effects of glucose, even in diabetic patients. This explains why hyperglycemic T2DM patients can utilize as much glucose as non-diabetic subjects at normoglycemia, despite their insulin resistance.

The degree of insulin resistance in T2DM patients is directly proportional to the severity of hyperglycemia. Insulin resistance induced through the hexosamine pathway in hyperglycemic T2DM patients can be seen as a compensatory mechanism to protect muscles from excessive glucose uptake.

The Hexosamine Pathway

Discovered in 1991 by Marshall et al., the hexosamine pathway mediates glucose-induced insulin resistance in primary cultured rat adipocytes. Downregulation of the insulin-responsive glucose transport system requires glucose, insulin, and glutamine. Inactivation of the enzyme glutamine: fructose-6-phosphate amidotransferase (GFA) by glutamine analogs prevents glucose-induced desensitization of glucose transport. GFA, expressed in insulin target tissues such as skeletal muscle, catalyzes the conversion of glutamine and fructose-6-phosphate to glucosamine-6-phosphate (GlcN-6-P) and glutamate. The pathway's end-product, UDP-N-acetylglucosamine (UDP-GlcNAc), results in O-glycation of proteins involved in glucose-responsive and insulin-dependent transcription and signaling events.

Causes of Insulin Resistance in Muscle

Obesity

Obesity reduces insulin-stimulated glucose uptake in skeletal muscle, independently of physical fitness changes. This reduction is partially attributed to increased NEFA from adipose tissue and fat accumulation in myocytes.

Abdominal Obesity

Insulin resistance in skeletal muscle is more severe in individuals with android (abdominal) obesity compared to those with gynoid obesity. Histologically, abdominally obese subjects show decreased capillary density and an insulin-resistant fiber type in their skeletal muscles.

Physical Inactivity

Sedentary lifestyles significantly contribute to obesity and T2DM. Several epidemiologic studies have demonstrated an inverse relationship between physical activity and T2DM incidence. Insulin sensitivity of glucose uptake by skeletal muscle is directly proportional to physical fitness, measured by maximal oxygen consumption (VO2max). Decreased physical fitness in T2DM patients is characterized by reduced capillary density and impaired mitochondrial oxidative phosphorylation. Resistive training improves glucose tolerance and insulin-stimulated glucose uptake by increasing total muscle mass.

Exercise and Insulin Resistance

Exercise and insulin stimulate glucose uptake through independent mechanisms. Insulin enhances glucose uptake via the classic insulin signaling pathway, whereas exercise activates adenosine 5'-monophosphate-activated protein kinase (AMPK), leading to GLUT-4 translocation to the cell membrane and increased glucose transport. In insulin-resistant T2DM patients, the ability of insulin to stimulate key signaling pathways is subnormal. However, aerobic training increases GLUT-4 content and glycogen synthase activity in skeletal muscle to levels comparable to normal subjects, indicating that exercise-enhanced glucose uptake pathways may remain intact in T2DM patients.

Metabolic Syndrome and Cardiovascular Risk

Insulin resistance is characterized by various abnormalities beyond glucose homeostasis, contributing to metabolic syndrome. This syndrome includes hypertriglyceridemia, low HDL cholesterol, small LDL size, hypertension, increased uric acid, and elevated PAI-1 levels, among other factors. Recognizing metabolic syndrome is crucial due to its association with preventable components of premature atherosclerosis and cardiovascular disease, the leading cause of mortality in T2DM patients. The accumulation of fat in the liver, independent of obesity, appears to be a significant factor in metabolic syndrome. Genetic and acquired factors contribute to fat accumulation in the liver, leading to increased cardiovascular risk.

Insulin resistance, present even in non-diabetic individuals, encompasses abnormalities in glucose homeostasis and several other metabolic dysfunctions, significantly contributing to cardiovascular risk in T2DM patients. Addressing these metabolic disturbances through improved glycemic control and lifestyle modifications is essential in managing and mitigating the adverse effects associated with insulin resistance and metabolic syndrome.

CHAPTER TEN
METABOLIC DISTURBANCES IN DIABETES

Key Points:
- Type 1 diabetes results from immune-mediated destruction of pancreatic islets, leading to insulin deficiency.
- Metabolic changes in type 1 diabetes are influenced by insulin deficiency interacting with factors like diet and exercise.
- Type 2 diabetes involves complex interactions of genetic and environmental factors affecting insulin secretion, action, and glucose effectiveness.

Hyperglycemia is the defining metabolic abnormality in diabetes, marking elevated fasting and/or post-prandial blood glucose levels. The underlying abnormalities causing hyperglycemia vary among different diabetes subgroups, challenging the conventional categorization into type 1 and type 2 diabetes based solely on insulin deficiency.

Type 1 Diabetes (T1DM)

Type 1 diabetes, or immune-mediated diabetes, is characterized by immune destruction of insulin-secreting β-cells in the pancreatic islets. This leads to absolute insulin deficiency, inadequate to prevent lipolysis during systemic illness or severe physical stress. Interestingly, obese patients with T1DM may exhibit metabolic patterns similar to those with long-standing T2DM, blurring the traditional distinctions between the two types.

Type 2 Diabetes (T2DM)

In type 2 diabetes, although the pancreas produces insulin, its secretion and levels are inadequate for prevailing glucose concentrations. T2DM is predominantly viewed as a disorder of insulin signaling exacerbated by factors such as poor diet, obesity, and lack of physical activity.

Carbohydrate Metabolism

Fasting State:

Glucose production in the fasting state primarily involves endogenous glucose release from the liver and kidneys. Glucose concentrations typically range from 4.5 to 5.5 mmol/L following an overnight fast in non-diabetic individuals.

Gluconeogenesis:

Approximately 50-60% of endogenous glucose production post-overnight fast is derived from gluconeogenesis. This process utilizes three-carbon precursors like lactate, alanine, and glycerol.

Insulin Effect:

Insulin plays a critical role in glucose metabolism. In the fasting state, insulin-independent glucose disposal occurs in tissues such as the brain, splanchnic tissues, and erythrocytes. Insulin-mediated glucose disposal primarily occurs in muscle, while low insulin levels lead to increased reliance on free fatty acids (FFA) for energy.

Postprandial State
Glucose Regulation:
After a meal, insulin secretion increases rapidly in response to rising glucose levels, suppressing glucagon secretion and enhancing hepatic glucose uptake. Splanchnic tissues initially extract glucose, with muscle accounting for the majority of glucose disposal, thus limiting post-prandial glucose elevation.

Impaired Fasting Glucose (IFG):
Studies suggest that impaired fasting glucose (IFG) is associated with decreased insulin action, increased endogenous glucose production, and hepatic insulin resistance. Individuals with IFG have a higher risk of progressing to type 2 diabetes within 5-10 years.

Insulin Resistance in Diabetes:
Both type 1 and type 2 diabetes involve insulin resistance, albeit in different forms. In type 1

diabetes, insulin action is tissue-specific, with cardiac muscle maintaining normal glucose uptake. Conversely, insulin binding in adipocytes may be decreased due to the metabolic milieu rather than an intrinsic defect.

Insulin plays a pivotal role in glucose metabolism, facilitating glucose uptake predominantly in muscles and suppressing EGP. Post-absorptive, insulin-independent glucose disposal occurs in the brain, splanchnic tissues, and erythrocytes. Conversely, low insulin levels in the postabsorptive state promote lipolysis and limit muscle glucose uptake. Postprandial insulin secretion promptly responds to rising glucose levels, enhancing glucose uptake and suppressing glucagon secretion to stabilize post-meal glucose levels.

Type 1 Diabetes (T1DM)
T1DM results from autoimmune destruction of pancreatic β-cells, leading to insulin deficiency. Even before clinical diabetes develops, affected individuals exhibit defects in insulin secretion

and action. Impaired insulin action primarily affects glucose uptake pathways, necessitating exogenous insulin to control glycemia effectively. Despite systemic hyperinsulinemia associated with subcutaneous insulin delivery, the benefits in glycemic control outweigh potential negative effects on insulin action.

Type 2 Diabetes (T2DM)
T2DM is characterized by elevated fasting and postprandial glucose levels due to impaired insulin secretion and action. Early abnormalities include delayed and decreased insulin secretion in response to food intake. Chronic hyperglycemia and elevated free fatty acids (FFA) levels further impair insulin secretion. Insulin resistance, notably in muscles and adipose tissues, exacerbates hyperglycemia by limiting glucose uptake and promoting hepatic glucose production.

Diabetes encompasses a spectrum of metabolic disorders influenced by genetic predisposition and environmental factors. Understanding the nuanced roles of insulin secretion, action, and glucose effectiveness is crucial for tailoring effective therapeutic strategies. Advances in pharmacotherapy, including agents targeting insulin secretion, action, and glucagon suppression, hold promise for optimizing glucose metabolism in diabetic individuals.

Insulin and Glucose Regulation in Lipid Metabolism

Adipose Tissue and Muscle LPL Activity

Insulin and glucose play critical roles in lipid metabolism by selectively stimulating lipoprotein lipase (LPL) activity in adipose tissue while inhibiting it in muscle. This mechanism directs triglycerides and lipoprotein-derived fatty acids towards adipose tissue rather than muscle. However, in type 2 diabetes mellitus (T2DM), the activation of adipose LPL by insulin is delayed, while skeletal muscle LPL activity is enhanced. This shift is significant because elevated free fatty acids

(FFAs) can further impair muscle glucose uptake, exacerbating insulin resistance. FFAs inhibit glucose transport, glucose phosphorylation, and muscle glycogen synthase, contributing to decreased glucose utilization in muscle tissue.

Protein Metabolism in Diabetes

Regulatory Factors

Protein synthesis and breakdown are regulated by substrate availability and hormonal balance, with insulin being a critical regulator. Significant changes in body composition can occur following the initiation of insulin therapy in individuals with type 1 diabetes mellitus (T1DM), particularly if insulin deficiency has been severe and prolonged. Urinary nitrogen excretion, a marker of protein metabolism, varies in response to changes in glucose production and severity of hyperglycemia. In T2DM, insulin-induced stimulation of splanchnic glucose uptake is impaired, largely due to decreased extracellular glucose uptake, suggesting lower glucokinase activity.

Lipid Metabolism in Diabetes

Triglyceride Dynamics

Triglycerides serve as a major energy source and storage form, mobilized as FFAs. FFAs are taken up and re-esterified in adipose and hepatic tissues or oxidized in muscle and liver. They are released through intravascular lipolysis of triglyceride-rich lipoproteins and intra-adipocyte lipolysis of triglyceride stores. In fasting states, FFA concentrations are primarily determined by their rate of entry into circulation, while in postprandial states, uptake by adipose and hepatic tissues also plays a significant role.

Hormonal Regulation of Lipolysis

Hormone-sensitive lipase, a key regulator of FFA release from adipose tissue, is highly sensitive to insulin. Insulin, the main hormonal regulator of lipolysis, inhibits lipolysis by increasing plasma glucose concentrations after meals, thereby suppressing FFA release. This suppression enhances insulin-dependent glucose disposal and inhibits endogenous glucose production. Conversely, falling blood glucose levels in non-diabetic individuals lead to increased lipolysis due to decreased insulin secretion, raising FFA levels to stabilize or increase glucose concentrations.

Insulin Deficiency and FFA Dynamics

In T1DM, absolute or relative insulin deficiency results in elevated FFAs, which impair peripheral glucose uptake and stimulate endogenous glucose production, contributing to increased ketogenesis and risk of ketoacidosis. Insulin counteracts the lipolytic effects of other hormones, such as growth hormone or cortisol, which have limited effects on lipolysis unless insulin availability is reduced. The lipolytic effect of catecholamines is also modulated by insulin levels, being blunted by hyperinsulinemia and accentuated by hypoinsulinemia. Although glucagon does not affect systemic FFA availability, its increased levels in uncontrolled diabetes can drive hepatic metabolism towards ketogenesis.

Exercise and FFA Availability

Moderate-intensity exercise typically results in decreased insulin and increased catecholamine concentrations, enhancing FFA availability and fatty acid oxidation. However, plasma insulin levels do not decrease with exercise, indicating a complex interplay between physical activity and metabolic regulation in diabetes.

Ketoacidosis and Its Triggers

Physical Stress and Hormonal Responses

Ketoacidosis, a serious complication in diabetes, is frequently triggered by physical stressors such as infections or surgical procedures. In the presence of insulin deficiency, glucagon levels rise, particularly during physical stress. Additionally, a reduction in effective circulating blood volume can elevate glucagon levels since glucagon is cleared by the kidneys. The concentrations of other counter-regulatory hormones also increase, further promoting lipolysis and exacerbating the condition.

Osmotic Diuresis and Electrolyte Imbalance

Both ketone bodies and glucose contribute to osmotic diuresis, which worsens hypovolemia and electrolyte imbalances caused by metabolic acidosis. Ketone bodies can also induce vomiting, leading to further electrolyte and fluid losses, directly contributing to metabolic acidosis. Severe acidosis can result in cardiovascular collapse. Intracellular metabolic acidosis disrupts several enzymatic processes, aggravating the effects of circulatory failure. Ultimately, death in ketoacidosis can be due to underlying comorbidities or the precipitating illness, such as myocardial infarction or pneumonia, or as a direct consequence of severe acidosis.

CHAPTER ELEVEN
OBESITY AND DIABETES

Key Points
- Definition and Prevalence: Obesity is defined by a body mass index (BMI) of 30 kg/m² or higher and is characterized by excess body fat. Its prevalence has risen significantly over recent decades, now affecting 15-30% of adults in Western countries.
- Risk Factor for T2DM: Overweight and obesity are the most significant modifiable risk factors for type 2 diabetes mellitus (T2DM). Abdominal fat distribution is closely associated with T2DM, particularly in individuals with lower BMIs.
- Genetic Influences: Both obesity and T2DM have strong genetic components. Obesity-related genes typically affect

central pathways of food intake, while T2DM risk genes primarily impair β-cell function.
- Environmental Contributors:Key environmental factors in obesity include high-calorie diets, large portion sizes, constant food availability, physical inactivity, and low socioeconomic status.
- Insulin Resistance:Increased adipose tissue in obesity impairs insulin action, causing insulin resistance in muscle, adipose tissue, liver, and possibly other organs.
- Inflammation and Cellular Dysfunction: Obesity is associated with subacute chronic inflammation in adipose tissue, mitochondrial dysfunction, local hypoxia, and other cellular disturbances.
- Weight Loss Benefits: Weight loss in obese individuals leads to rapid improvement in metabolic disturbances, including chronic inflammation and insulin resistance. These benefits arise

from caloric restriction rather than specific macronutrient compositions.
- Bariatric Surgery: Bariatric surgery is the most effective treatment for morbid obesity and can significantly improve or even resolve metabolic disturbances, including T2DM.

Obesity, a chronic disorder characterized by excessive body fat, has become a global epidemic affecting industrialized, developing, and underdeveloped countries. Currently, obesity (BMI $\geq$ 30 kg/m²) affects 15-30% of adults in Europe, North America, and many Arabic countries, with a clear trend of increasing prevalence. Obesity increases the risk of numerous health issues, including metabolic disturbances like T2DM, cardiovascular complications, locomotor disorders, and various cancers. Additionally, obesity reduces life expectancy and impairs quality of life. The close relationship between excessive body weight and diabetes risk highlights the broader health impacts of obesity.

Definition and Body Fat Distribution

Obesity diagnosis and classification are primarily based on BMI, calculated from body weight and height. BMI is categorized as follows by the World Health Organization (WHO):

- Underweight: <18.5 kg/m²
- Normal weight: 18.5-24.9 kg/m²
- Overweight: ≥25 kg/m²
- Obesity:
  - Grade I: 30-34.9 kg/m²
  - Grade II: 35-39.9 kg/m²
  - Grade III: ≥40 kg/m²

In Western countries, 30-50% of the population is classified as overweight (BMI 25-29.9 kg/m²). The distribution of body fat, particularly abdominal fat, significantly affects metabolic risk. Abdominal fat distribution increases diabetes risk even in individuals with a BMI in the upper normal range. Therefore, waist circumference should be routinely measured to assess diabetes risk.

Obesity as a Risk Factor for T2DM

Extensive clinical data show a strong correlation between body fat mass and diabetes risk. Unlike other obesity-associated metabolic issues, diabetes risk increases even in the upper normal BMI range. For example, women with a BMI of 23.0-24.9 kg/m² have a four- to five-fold increased risk of developing diabetes compared to women with a BMI of <22 kg/m². Weight gain also predicts diabetes risk; for instance, women who gained 11.0-19.9 kg after age 18 had a significantly higher risk of developing diabetes.

Genetic Factors and Obesity

Obesity and T2DM have significant genetic influences. Mutations affecting the leptin-melanocortin signaling pathway are linked to early-onset obesity, particularly in children.

Functional mutations in the melanocortin-4 receptor gene are a common cause of monogenic obesity, accounting for 2-4% of all obesity cases in children.

Notably, these defects impact genes involved in the central regulation of food intake. Recent genome-wide association (GWA) studies in large cohorts with BMI as a phenotype have identified common genetic variants across various chromosomes. These obesity-predisposing polymorphisms are primarily associated with central food intake pathways. Consequently, human obesity may be seen as a heritable neurobehavioral disorder that is highly influenced by environmental conditions, especially in societies with abundant, energy-dense palatable foods. Despite significant advances in understanding the genetic factors contributing to obesity, the effect size of most identified "obesity genes" remains modest. For instance, individuals homozygous for the high-risk allele of the FTO gene weigh, on average, 3 kg more than those with two low-risk alleles.

Genetic Predisposition for Obesity and Type 2 Diabetes

It is well-established from family, adoption, and twin studies that obesity, like type 2 diabetes mellitus (T2DM), has a strong genetic basis. Stunkard et al.'s classic adoption study showed no correlation between the adult BMI of adopted Danish children and that of their adoptive parents, but a significant correlation with the BMI of their biological parents, particularly the biological mother. Twin studies have demonstrated that concordance rates for different degrees of overweight are twice as high for monozygotic twins compared to dizygotic twins, indicating high heritability for BMI at both 20 years of age and at a 25-year follow-up. This suggests substantial genetic control over body fatness. Furthermore, a study of 5092 twins in London estimated the heritability of BMI and waist circumference to be 0.77, reinforcing the significant impact of genetic components irrespective of the obesogenic environment. Recent discoveries of several monogenic disorders leading to human obesity have added to this understanding.

Environmental Factors Advancing Type 2 Diabetes and Obesity

A complex gene-environment interaction determines an individual's risk of developing obesity. In societies with an abundance of affordable, highly palatable food, body weight varies widely among individuals, from lean to extremely obese. Factors such as physical activity, education, and socioeconomic status also strongly influence body weight. Recent data from the USA and other Western countries suggest that after two to three decades of modern lifestyle, the trend toward obesity is plateauing, supporting the concept that genetic and biological factors significantly contribute to obesity susceptibility.

Despite genetic predispositions, the global obesity epidemic is widely recognized as a consequence of dramatic lifestyle and environmental changes over the past 30-50 years. Eating habits and food selections have shifted significantly, while physical activity has decreased due to technological advancements in transportation and workplaces. Both dietary abundance and sedentary lifestyles contribute to a chronic positive energy balance, resulting in energy storage in adipose tissue.

The rise of the fast-food culture, characterized by high-fat, low-starch foods and high consumption of sugar-sweetened beverages, is a novel phenomenon. Fast-food menus often have large portion sizes and high energy density, which is believed to contribute to weight gain and the maintenance of overweight and obesity. A recent systematic review of six cross-sectional and seven prospective cohort studies confirmed a significant association between frequent fast-food consumption and increased body weight, at least in adults. Moreover, a high intake of sugar-sweetened beverages is another aspect of the global fast-food culture contributing to obesity. Another systematic review concluded that high consumption of these beverages is a significant determinant of increased caloric intake.

Another factor in the obesity epidemic is the trend toward increasing portion sizes over the last few decades. A study in the USA showed that the average portion size for many foods increased markedly between 1977 and 1998, particularly for foods consumed at fast-food restaurants and at home. Other countries have also noticed similar tendencies. Experimental studies have clearly established that larger portion sizes and higher energy density of foods are associated with increased caloric intake, promoting weight gain and obesity over time.

Socioeconomic status is a strong determinant of obesity and T2DM. There is a gradient between education, household income, and obesity prevalence in most countries. Low socioeconomic status is associated with an unfavorable lifestyle, including poor nutrition, low physical activity, and low health consciousness. This gradient is usually more pronounced in females than in males. The association between low household income and obesity may be mediated by the low cost of energy-dense foods, whereas healthy diets based on lean meats, fish, vegetables, and fruit are less affordable for individuals with lower socioeconomic status.

Pathophysiological Links Between Obesity and Type 2 Diabetes

Type 2 diabetes mellitus (T2DM) is characterized by impaired insulin action or defective insulin secretion, or both. These defects are present many years before the clinical onset of the disease. While the mechanisms by which obesity increases the risk of developing T2DM are not fully understood, significant progress has been made in understanding how excessive fat mass and chronic overnutrition can cause metabolic disturbances leading to T2DM in genetically predisposed individuals.

The earliest hypothesis to explain the relationship between obesity and T2DM is the "glucose-fatty acid cycle," which posits a competition between glucose and fatty acid oxidation in the muscle. This hypothesis was introduced by Randle et al., who observed that an increased supply of non-esterified fatty acids from expanded adipose tissue depots competes with glucose utilization, particularly in muscle, reducing the rate of glucose oxidation and increasing glucose concentrations. Elevated free fatty acids can directly impair insulin action, with obese individuals and those with T2DM showing high intramyocellular lipid accumulation, a feature of the insulin-resistant state.

In addition to glucose, long-chain fatty acids can stimulate insulin secretion from pancreatic β-cells via fatty acyl CoA generation and protein kinase C activation. However, chronic exposure of β-cells to excessive fatty acids is associated with impaired glucose-stimulated insulin secretion and decreased insulin biosynthesis. Elevated fatty acids may also impair insulin secretion via increased expression of uncoupling protein 2 (UCP-2) in β-cells.

Adipose tissue is now recognized as a secretory organ producing various factors that contribute to insulin resistance and other health risks. Tumor necrosis factor-α (TNF-α), a multifunctional cytokine, was the first such factor identified in adipose tissue. TNF-α inhibits glucose uptake, reduces lipoprotein lipase expression, increases lipolysis, and activates the NF-κB pathway, leading to increased expression of proinflammatory proteins such as interleukin-6 (IL-6) and monocyte chemotactic protein-1 (MCP-1). Other adipokines, such as leptin, adiponectin, and resistin, also play significant roles in metabolism and energy homeostasis.

Recent studies have shown that defective mitochondrial function could be a prominent feature of disturbances in both insulin secretion and action, further complicating the relationship between obesity and T2DM.

Adipocytes also secrete anti-inflammatory agents such as adiponectin, IL-1 receptor antagonist, and IL-10. Adiponectin, notably the most abundant protein in adipose tissue, has been extensively studied and is inversely related to BMI, with lower levels predicting the onset of type 2 diabetes mellitus (T2DM). Adiponectin is known for its antidiabetic and anti-atherosclerotic effects, including the stimulation of fatty acid oxidation through an AMP-activated protein kinase-dependent pathway .

Signaling Pathways of Inflammation in Adipose Tissue

Current research indicates that inflammation in human obesity is mediated by the activation of the c-Jun N-terminal kinase (JNK) and IKKβ-NF-κB pathways. These pathways are triggered by cytokines like TNF-α and IL-6 as well as lipids. Experimental studies have shown that genetic or chemical inhibition of these pathways can reduce inflammation and improve insulin resistance . Elevated JNK activity is observed not only in adipose tissue but also in the liver and muscle in obesity. JNK1 loss prevents insulin resistance and diabetes in both genetic and dietary mouse models of obesity . IKKβ influences insulin signaling through phosphorylation of IRS-1 on serine residues and activation of NF-κB, promoting the production of pro-inflammatory mediators like TNF-α and IL-6 . Mice heterozygous for IKKβ show partial protection against lipid-induced insulin resistance . Both JNK and IKKβ-NF-κB pathways are activated via pattern recognition receptors responding to various signals, including endogenous lipids that activate toll-like receptors (TLRs).

Adipose Tissue Hypoxia

The expansion of adipose tissue mass leads to hypertrophy of fat cells and subsequent tissue hypoxia. Studies suggest that hypoxia plays a significant role in chronic inflammation, macrophage infiltration, impaired adipokine secretion, ER stress, and mitochondrial dysfunction in obesity. These effects are associated with inhibited adipogenesis, triglyceride synthesis, and elevated free fatty acid levels. Reduced interstitial partial oxygen pressure (PO_2) in obese adipose tissue has been documented, with PO_2 dropping by up to 70% compared to lean controls. Hypoxia also reduces mitochondrial respiration, increasing lactate production, and decreases adiponectin expression in adipocytes. The hypoxic state is linked to reduced blood flow and capillary density in adipose tissue, which persists despite increased production of pro-angiogenic factors like VEGF.

Accumulation of Immune Cells

Leptin, TNF-α, MCP-1, and other chemokines are crucial for recruiting macrophages to adipose tissue. The secretory profile of preadipocytes and adipocytes includes various chemoattractants for immune cells. Initial attraction of T-lymphocytes by stromal cell-derived factor 1 (SDF-1) leads to the invasion and activation of monocytes/macrophages . This immune cell accumulation and inflammation are more pronounced in omental than subcutaneous adipose tissue, aligning with the concept that visceral fat contributes significantly to metabolic and cardiovascular complications of obesity .

Role of Body Fat Distribution

Body fat distribution significantly affects metabolic and cardiovascular risk. Visceral adipose tissue, more metabolically active than subcutaneous fat, exhibits a higher expression of pro-inflammatory factors and greater immune cell accumulation. This tissue drains into the portal vein, directly exposing the liver to fatty acids and proteins, thereby promoting insulin resistance in the liver. Consequently, inflammation extends beyond adipose tissue to affect the liver and other organs.

Obesity and Endoplasmic Reticulum Stress

Obesity and chronic overnutrition overwhelm the endoplasmic reticulum (ER), causing ER stress and activating inflammatory signaling pathways, including JNK. In high-fat diet-induced and genetic obesity models, ER stress plays a critical role in insulin receptor signaling through IRE-1α-mediated JNK activation. Overexpression of the molecular chaperone ORP150 in a mouse model of type 2 diabetes improved insulin sensitivity and glucose uptake .

Treatment of Obesity in the Context of Metabolic Syndrome and Type 2 Diabetes

Obesity is a significant driver of T2DM, making weight management a crucial treatment strategy. Weight loss effectively prevents T2DM and improves metabolic disturbances in affected individuals. Studies indicate that modest to moderate weight loss significantly reduces pro-inflammatory factors like leptin, CRP, PAI-1, IL-6, IL-8, and MCP-1, while increasing adiponectin levels. Surgical weight loss in morbidly obese patients also reduces macrophage infiltration in adipose tissue .

Despite advancements, treating obese patients with type 2 diabetes mellitus (T2DM) remains more challenging than managing obesity alone. This is partly because individuals with T2DM tend to be older, resulting in lower energy expenditure and smaller weight loss. Additionally, these patients often prioritize blood glucose control, potentially neglecting other health issues. The weight gain or lack of weight loss associated with various antidiabetic medications also complicates treatment.

Dietary Approaches

Effective weight management in obese patients with T2DM requires a moderately hypocaloric diet, increased physical activity, and behavior modification, similar to recommendations for non-diabetic obese individuals. Numerous studies have explored these methods, critically evaluating their outcomes. The gold standard involves a balanced, moderately energy-restricted diet with an energy deficit of at least 500 kcal/day, emphasizing reduced fat intake, particularly saturated fats. A low-fat, high-carbohydrate diet is generally recommended, although some clinical studies suggest that replacing saturated fats with monounsaturated fats might offer additional benefits for glucose metabolism.

Weight-Lowering Drugs

Adjunctive use of weight-lowering drugs can be considered when non-pharmacologic treatments are insufficient. Current options include orlistat, a gastric and pancreatic lipase inhibitor, and GLP-1 mimetics like exenatide. Orlistat has shown to result in greater weight loss and slight improvements in HbA1c levels compared to placebo. GLP-1 mimetics, on the other hand, significantly promote weight loss in a high proportion of patients.

Bariatric Surgery

Bariatric surgery is increasingly recognized as an effective method for significant weight reduction in patients with T2DM and a BMI ≥ 35 kg/m². Long-term results from studies, such as the Swedish Obese Subjects study, indicate that surgical interventions not only achieve substantial weight loss but also reduce the incidence of T2DM and overall mortality. A meta-analysis of bariatric surgery outcomes in T2DM patients found that 78% achieved complete remission of diabetes, with the most effective results seen in combined restrictive and malabsorptive procedures.

Therefore, Obesity significantly increases the risk of developing T2DM due to its impact on insulin resistance and secretion. Thus, weight management is crucial for improving metabolic control in T2DM patients. Although conventional approaches combining diet and physical activity often yield poor long-term results, there is a need for developing and evaluating more effective weight loss strategies.

CHAPTER TWELVE
MONOGENIC CAUSES OF DIABETES

Key Points

Monogenic diabetes which results from mutations in a single gene leading to β-cell dysfunction or, less commonly, insulin resistance.
- Prevalence: Monogenic diabetes accounts for about 1-2% of diabetes cases but is often misdiagnosed.
- Indicators: Consider monogenic diabetes in atypical presentations for type 1 or 2 diabetes, in cases with an autosomal dominant family history (or maternally inherited mitochondrial disorders), characteristic features such as deafness in mitochondrial diabetes, fat loss in lipodystrophy, or diagnosis within the first six months of life.
- Glucokinase gene mutations: These mutations, important for glucose sensing in the pancreas,

reset fasting glucose levels to 5.5-8.0 mmol/L. Patients exhibit mild fasting hyperglycemia with minor changes in glycated hemoglobin and rarely require treatment.

- Transcription factor gene mutations (HNF1A, HNF4A): These mutations cause dominantly inherited progressive hyperglycemia, leading to symptomatic diabetes in adolescence or young adulthood. Patients are highly responsive to sulfonylurea treatment and may not need insulin until middle or old age.

- Mitochondrial mutations: These result in maternally inherited diabetes, often accompanied by sensorineural hearing loss and various other disorders.

- Early-onset diabetes: Diabetes diagnosed before six months is unlikely to be type 1 and warrants genetic testing. High-dose sulfonylurea treatment may be more effective than insulin for mutations in Kir6.2 and SUR1 subunits of the β-cell potassium channel.

- Insulin resistance indicators: Acanthosis nigricans in non-obese patients suggest a genetic cause. Partial lipodystrophy, indicating thin muscular limbs with hypertriglyceridemia and insulin resistance, suggests a mutation in LMNA or PPARG. In the absence of lipodystrophy, an insulin receptor mutation is the most common cause.

Monogenic diabetes arises from mutations in a single gene and constitutes 1-2% of all diabetes cases. These mutations can be inherited in either a dominant or recessive manner. The majority of monogenic diabetes cases (90%) are initially misclassified as type 1 or type 2 diabetes. Accurate genetic diagnosis is crucial for predicting clinical outcomes, explaining associated clinical features, providing genetic counseling, diagnosing family members, and guiding appropriate treatment.

Monogenic diabetes affecting the β-cell primarily presents in four ways: familial mild fasting hyperglycemia (glucokinase maturity-onset diabetes of the young [MODY]), familial young-onset diabetes (transcription factor MODY), neonatal diabetes, and diabetes with extrapancreatic features. Clinical and biochemical characteristics that distinguish common forms of monogenic diabetes from type 1 and type 2 diabetes are summarized in Table below.

Table: 13.1

Characteristic	Type 1 Diabetes Type 2 Diabetes	Type 2 Diabetes	Monogenic Diabetes
Age of Onset	Usually <30 years	Usually >40 years	Often <25 years, but can vary
Family History	Often absent	Often present	Strong family history, autosomal dominant
Autoantibodies	Present (e.g., GAD, IA2, ZnT8)	Absent	Absent

C-Peptide Levels	Low or undetectable	Normal or high	Usually detectable, but can be low
Body Mass Index (BMI)	Often normal or underweight	Often overweight or obese	Varies, but often normal
Insulin Resistance	Low	High	Low to moderate
Insulin Requirement	Yes, lifelong	Yes, progressive need	Varies, some forms may not require insulin
Genetic Testing	Not typically performed	Not typically performed	Diagnostic, identifies specific mutations
Response	Poor	Good	Varies,

to Oral Agents			some forms respond well
DKA at Diagnosis	Common	Rare	Rare
Treatment Focus	Insulin therapy	Lifestyle changes, oral meds	Tailored to specific mutation
Example Subtypes	N/A	N/A	MODY, Neonatal diabetes, others

Notes:

MODY (Maturity Onset Diabetes of the Young) is a common form of monogenic diabetes that often presents with mild hyperglycemia and can be managed with sulfonylureas or other oral agents instead of insulin. Neonatal diabetes presents within the first six months of life and may be transient or permanent. Genetic testing is critical in monogenic diabetes for accurate diagnosis and tailored treatment.

Maturity-Onset Diabetes of the Young (MODY)

MODY is an autosomal dominantly inherited form of diabetes that occurs in young individuals but is not insulin-dependent. In lieu of insulin resistance, it is caused by β-cell malfunction. Genetic etiologies have been identified, allowing MODY to be subclassified according to the involved gene. Mutations in at least eight genes have been linked to MODY, including those encoding the glucose-sensing enzyme glucokinase (GCK) and several transcription factors affecting β-cell development and function. Table 13.1 provides a summary of the clinical features of glucokinase and transcription factor diabetes. Due to the diverse subtypes of MODY, defining the genetic etiology is essential. We recommend categorizing based on the genetic cause: familial mild fasting hyperglycemia from GCK mutations (GCK MODY), familial young-onset progressive diabetes from HNF1A and HNF4A mutations (transcription factor MODY), and renal cysts and diabetes syndrome (RCAD) from HNF1B mutations.

Genetic testing for MODY should be considered in patients diagnosed with diabetes before the age of 25, who do not fully match the phenotypes of type 1 or type 2 diabetes, and have a strong family history of diabetes. Differentiation from type 1 diabetes is crucial as these patients can often be managed effectively without insulin.

Glucokinase MODY

Glucokinase catalyzes the phosphorylation of glucose to glucose-6-phosphate, the first and rate-limiting step in intracellular glucose metabolism in both β-cells and hepatocytes. This process allows β-cells and hepatocytes to respond to changes in glucose levels. In β-cells, glucokinase functions as a glucose sensor, ensuring insulin release is appropriate for the glucose concentration. Heterozygous loss-of-function mutations in GCK shift the dose-response curve to the right, resulting in regulated but elevated glycemia. Over 200 loss-of-function mutations in GCK have been identified, all presenting similarly. Homozygous loss-of-function mutations cause neonatal insulin-requiring diabetes, while gain-of-function mutations lead to congenital hyperinsulinism.

Patients with GCK mutations exhibit mild fasting hyperglycemia from birth, usually between 5.5-8.0 mmol/L, with minimal glycemic deterioration over time. They are generally asymptomatic, with postprandial glucose levels mildly elevated and near-normal HbA1c values, explaining the rarity of complications.

Differentiating from Type 1 and 2 Diabetes

Diagnosing glucokinase MODY is particularly important in young patients who might otherwise be misdiagnosed with type 1 diabetes and unnecessarily treated with insulin. Unlike type 1 diabetes, hyperglycemia in glucokinase MODY is mild, β-cell antibodies are typically negative, and one parent is likely to have mild hyperglycemia. Fasting C-peptide remains detectable, and postprandial glucose increments are less pronounced than in type 1 diabetes. Distinguishing glucokinase MODY from type 2 diabetes can be more challenging, as both conditions can exhibit mild hyperglycemia with a strong family history. Absence of obesity, lack of insulin resistance, minimal oral glucose tolerance test increments, and non-progression are indicative of glucokinase MODY.

Management

Outside of pregnancy, hypoglycemic medication is generally unnecessary for glucokinase MODY due to the mild nature of hyperglycemia and the rarity of complications. Once the diagnosis is confirmed, treatment can usually be discontinued, but caution is advised as type 1 or type 2 diabetes can coexist with a GCK mutation. Monitoring for significant changes in glycemia is important, as this may indicate the development of type 1 or type 2 diabetes in addition to the GCK mutation.

Transcription Factors and MODY

Transcription factors are proteins that bind to DNA, playing a crucial role in the regulatory network that governs gene expression. Most patients with Maturity Onset Diabetes of the Young (MODY) have a heterozygous mutation in a transcription factor gene, with the most common mutations found in hepatic nuclear factors HNF1A and HNF4A. Other transcription factors involved in MODY include HNF1B, insulin promoter factor 1 (IPF-1), and NEUROD1.

Clinical Features

Heterozygous mutations in transcription factors cause autosomal dominant diabetes, typically presenting in adolescence or early adulthood due to progressive insulin secretion failure. While diabetes manifestations are similar in carriers of HNF1A and HNF4A mutations due to common patterns of β-cell dysfunction, there are distinct differences in extrapancreatic features.

Glucokinase MODY and Pregnancy

Patients with GCK mutations often present with hyperglycemia detected during pregnancy screening, representing around 3% of Caucasian patients with gestational diabetes. Identifying these mutations is crucial as they dictate a different clinical course compared to other forms of gestational diabetes. The birth weight of the newborn depends on the mutation status of both the mother and the fetus. If only the mother carries the mutation, maternal hyperglycemia can lead to increased fetal insulin secretion and growth, resulting in a larger fetus. Conversely, if the fetus inherits the mutation from the father, birth weight is reduced due to lower fetal insulin secretion and growth.

Genetic Testing for GCK Mutations in Pregnancy

Testing for GCK mutations is recommended when a pregnant patient exhibits persistent fasting plasma glucose levels of 5.5–8 mmol/L and an increment of less than 4.6 mmol/L on an oral glucose tolerance test. A lack of family history should not exclude the diagnosis, as asymptomatic hyperglycemia in a parent might go undetected.

Management

Patients with hyperglycemia due to glucokinase mutations are often treated with insulin during pregnancy to manage fasting hyperglycemia. However, the fetal genotype is a more significant determinant of birth weight than maternal treatment, as insulin therapy appears to have minimal effect on fetal growth.

Differentiating from Type 1 and Type 2 Diabetes

Patients with MODY are frequently misdiagnosed with Type 1 Diabetes Mellitus (T1DM) due to symptomatic diabetes in adolescence or early adulthood. Genetic testing for HNF1A mutations is recommended for young adults with presumed T1DM, a family history of diabetes, and negative antibody tests at diagnosis. Features suggestive of MODY include the absence of ketosis without insulin treatment, good glycemic control on low insulin doses, or detectable C-peptide levels with plasma glucose above 8 mmol/L three to five years post-diagnosis. Positive GAD antibodies may not exclude monogenic diabetes, especially in cases with high clinical suspicion.

For suspected Type 2 Diabetes Mellitus (T2DM) patients, HNF1A mutations should be considered if there is young-onset diabetes (before age 25 in at least one family member), a strong family history of diabetes (particularly in non-obese individuals diagnosed in their twenties or thirties), and a lack of obesity or other insulin resistance markers. Supporting features include a large increment in glucose tolerance tests, glycosuria with blood glucose less than 10 mmol/L, marked sensitivity to sulfonylureas, and atypical lipid profiles (normal or raised HDL and normal or low triglycerides).

Management in Pregnancy

For pregnant patients with HNF1A and HNF4A mutations, sulfonylurea therapy is typically continued if glycemic control was good before pregnancy. If necessary, insulin treatment is initiated. Consideration should be given to switching to glibenclamide before pregnancy due to its established safety profile. If the fetus carries an HNF4A mutation, there is a significant risk of macrosomia and neonatal hypoglycemia, regardless of whether the mutation is inherited from the mother or father.

Early delivery may be considered if macrosomia is detected.

Neonatal Diabetes

Children diagnosed with diabetes within the first six months of life, known as neonatal diabetes, are likely to have monogenic diabetes rather than T1DM. Neonatal diabetes is rare, affecting 1 in 100,000 to 200,000 live births, and can present with ketoacidosis and absent C-peptide. Approximately half of these cases remit spontaneously and are termed transient neonatal diabetes mellitus (TNDM), while the rest persist as permanent neonatal diabetes mellitus (PNDM). Genetic mutations in key β-cell development or function genes are responsible for neonatal diabetes.

Management

Patients with HNF1A and HNF4A mutations respond well to sulfonylurea therapy, which is recommended as the first-line treatment.

Glycemic control with sulfonylureas is often superior to insulin, and the glucose-lowering effect is more pronounced than in T2DM. However, low doses may cause hypoglycemia, so starting doses should be conservative. For those with cardiovascular risk, statin therapy is advised for all patients over 40.

Transient Neonatal Diabetes

Over 90% of transient neonatal diabetes cases have a known genetic cause, predominantly linked to abnormalities in the 6q24 region of chromosome 6 affecting imprinted genes. These can be inherited or sporadic, with most cases involving mutations in KCNJ11 and ABCC8.

T cell antibodies are typically negative, and C-peptide levels are low or negligible. Low birth weight is common, averaging 2.1 kg, with potential accompanying conditions such as macroglossia or umbilical hernia. Insulin treatment is generally required for a median of 12 weeks before remission occurs. Diabetes recurs later in life in 50-60% of patients due to β-cell dysfunction, with an average recurrence age of 14 years. In some cases, hyperglycemia may be intermittent, appearing only during stress. For TNDM caused by KCNJ11 and ABCC8 mutations, diabetes typically presents later (median 4 weeks), takes longer to remit, and is associated with less intrauterine growth restriction (median birth weight 2.6 kg)

Management

Insulin is required during the neonatal period, whereas treatment requirements after relapse can range from dietary management to oral hypoglycemics or insulin. For TNDM due to KCNJ11 and ABCC8 mutations, diabetes may be successfully managed with sulfonylureas.

Genetic Counseling

The risk of recurrence in siblings or offspring depends on the genetic etiology. Cases caused by uniparental disomy are sporadic with a low recurrence risk. Methylation defects, often resulting from homozygous mutations in the transcription factor gene ZFP57, can be inherited in an autosomal recessive manner. Offspring of males with 6q24 duplication have a 50% chance of developing TNDM, whereas maternal inheritance does not affect the immediate generation but may affect subsequent generations.

Genetic Testing in Neonatal Diabetes

At diagnosis, it is unclear whether neonatal diabetes will be transient or permanent. Testing for 6q24 abnormalities, KCNJ11, ABCC8, and INS mutations is recommended for all diabetes cases diagnosed before 6 months. Identifying these mutations is crucial for determining treatment. An early diagnosis and very low birth weight suggest a high likelihood of 6q24 involvement. A genetic cause can be established in approximately 7% of diabetes cases diagnosed between 6 months and 1 year, warranting consideration for testing in this age group, especially when autoantibody tests are negative.

Diabetes with Extrapancreatic Features

Several monogenic diabetes forms are associated with extrapancreatic features. These may include renal cysts, exocrine pancreatic deficiency, genitourinary abnormalities, neurosensory deafness, and other systemic conditions.

Maternally Inherited Diabetes and Deafness (MIDD)

MIDD results from a mitochondrial DNA mutation causing maternally inherited diabetes with sensorineural deafness and potentially other features. It affects up to 1% of diabetes patients but is often undiagnosed.

Clinical Features

Most mutation carriers develop diabetes (over 85%) and sensorineural hearing loss (over 75%). Diabetes is progressive and typically presents insidiously like T2DM but can also present acutely with ketoacidosis in about 8% of cases.

The mean age of diabetes diagnosis is 37 years, but it can range from early adolescence to old age.

Pathogenesis

The m.3243A>G point mutation in mitochondrial DNA is the primary cause of mitochondrial diabetes, affecting the mitochondrial respiratory chain and potentially causing cellular energy deficiency. This impacts organs with high metabolic activity, including the endocrine pancreas, cochlea, retina, muscle, kidney, and brain. Mitochondrial dysfunction in pancreatic islets leads to abnormal β-cell function and insulin deficiency, while insulin sensitivity usually remains normal or slightly reduced. As mitochondria are maternally inherited, the maternal line is affected, and children of a male patient are not at risk. Phenotypic variation within a family is due to heteroplasmy.

Differentiating from Type 1 and 2 Diabetes

Diabetes caused by the m.3243A>G mutation may resemble T1DM or T2DM. GAD antibodies are usually negative. The presence of deafness or a family history of diabetes or deafness on the maternal side should prompt testing for the m.3243A>G mutation. Additional symptoms such as short stature, early-onset cardiomyopathy, myopathy, early-onset stroke, or macular retinal dystrophy may suggest MIDD.

Management

Early insulin treatment is typically required (mean 2 years post-diagnosis). Metformin is generally avoided due to the risk of lactic acidosis. Coenzyme Q10 supplementation may offer benefits, although further trials are needed. Monitoring for cardiac issues from a young age is recommended, particularly if there is a family history of early cardiomyopathy. Aggressive blood pressure management and early ACE inhibitor treatment may be appropriate due to the high risk of renal complications. Renal biopsy to exclude FSGS may be necessary in cases of renal failure. Hearing loss management includes avoiding exacerbating factors, prompt treatment of ear infections, hearing aids, and potentially cochlear implants for profound hearing loss.

Renal Cysts and Diabetes (HNF1B MODY)

HNF1B is a transcription factor involved in gene regulation in the pancreas, kidneys, liver, genital tract, and gut. Heterozygous deletions or mutations in HNF1B can cause developmental abnormalities, with renal abnormalities and diabetes being the most common. HNF1B abnormalities may be inherited in an autosomal dominant manner, but 32-58% of cases arise spontaneously.

Clinical Features

The clinical features include developmental renal disease, often manifested as renal cysts, with other possible renal abnormalities such as glomerulocystic kidney disease and cystic renal dysplasia. Half of the mutation carriers have early-onset diabetes due to both insulin deficiency from reduced β-cell number and increased hepatic insulin resistance. Sensitivity to sulfonylureas, seen in other transcription factor diabetes, is absent in HNF1B-related diabetes.

Differentiating from Type 1 and 2 Diabetes

About 50% of HNF1B mutations and deletions are spontaneous, and patients may not have a family history. Testing for HNF1B abnormalities should be considered in cases of unexplained cystic renal disease or other renal developmental abnormalities, with or without a past medical or family history of diabetes. It should also be considered for individuals with genital tract abnormalities associated with renal abnormalities. Testing should include dosage analysis to detect gene deletions, as these are common and may be missed if only sequencing is performed.

Management

Early insulin therapy is typically required for managing diabetes. Sulfonylurea sensitivity seen in other transcription factor diabetes is absent in HNF1B-related diabetes. Renal management is similar to other chronic progressive renal diseases. We recommend repeating renal ultrasound imaging every two years due to the potential increased risk of chromophobe renal carcinoma and annual diabetes screening in non-diabetic mutation carriers.

Inherited Subtypes of Lipodystrophy

Familial Partial Lipodystrophy

Familial partial lipodystrophies are autosomal dominant disorders characterized by the loss of subcutaneous fat in specific body regions. The primary subtypes are linked to mutations in the LMNA and PPARG genes.

LMNA Mutation (Dunnigan Lipodystrophy): This subtype leads to a gradual loss of subcutaneous fat from the limbs starting at puberty, often accompanied by muscle hypertrophy, giving a muscular appearance to the arms and legs. Fat loss may also occur in the anterior abdomen and chest, while excess fat is deposited in the face, neck, and intra-abdominal regions. Women with this condition commonly develop diabetes and hypertriglyceridemia, which can lead to pancreatitis. Acanthosis nigricans and polycystic ovarian syndrome are less common, and while hepatic steatosis is possible, cirrhosis is rare. There is a significant risk of cardiovascular mortality.

PPARG Mutation: This form shares phenotypic similarities with the LMNA mutation but tends to present more frequently with hypertension. Diagnosing this condition in women is usually straightforward, but it can be more challenging in men due to the muscular appearance of the limbs. The presence of early-onset diabetes in non-obese patients with hypertriglyceridemia should prompt consideration of lipodystrophy, especially if there is significant peripheral fat loss.

Congenital Generalized Lipodystrophy (Berardinelli-Seip Syndrome)

This rare autosomal recessive disorder is marked by an almost complete absence of subcutaneous fat from birth, giving affected individuals a muscular appearance. Due to the lack of functional adipocytes, lipids are stored in metabolically active tissues, leading to severe insulin resistance. Common features include widespread acanthosis, hypertriglyceridemia, low HDL cholesterol, and early-onset hepatic steatosis, which can progress to cirrhosis.

Three molecularly distinct forms have been identified: congenital generalized lipodystrophy types 1, 2, and 3, resulting from mutations in the AGPAT2, BSCL2, and CAV1 genes, respectively. Types 1 and 2 account for most cases, with some phenotypic differences.

However, some patients do not have mutations in these genes, suggesting other genetic etiologies remain undiscovered.

Other Inherited Forms of Lipodystrophy

Other rare forms of lipodystrophy include mandibuloacral dysplasia (characterized by skeletal abnormalities), SHORT syndrome (characterized by short stature, hyperextensible joints, ocular depression, Reiger anomaly, and delayed teething), and neonatal progeroid syndrome.

Management of Lipodystrophy

Management focuses on addressing insulin resistance and associated complications, such as diabetes, cardiovascular and cerebrovascular diseases, recurrent pancreatitis, cirrhosis, and psychological distress related to appearance.

Lifestyle Modifications: Patients are advised to follow a very low-fat diet (less than 15% of total energy from fat) and increase physical activity. Persistent hypertriglyceridemia and uncontrolled hyperglycemia may necessitate treatment with fibrates and high doses of fish oils. Estrogen replacement, including contraceptive pills, may worsen hypertriglyceridemia and is generally avoided.

Glycemic Control: This often requires a combination of oral medications and high-dose insulin. Metformin is commonly used to improve insulin sensitivity, although there is limited trial data for inherited lipodystrophies. Thiazolidinediones show variable effectiveness. Insulin requirements can be very high, with U500 insulin being appropriate in some cases. If proteinuric renal disease develops, a low threshold for renal biopsy is recommended due to the higher prevalence of non-diabetic renal diseases in these patients.

Leptin Replacement Therapy: Given the marked reduction in leptin levels in severe lipodystrophies, leptin replacement has shown significant improvements in glycemic control and hypertriglyceridemia, and it may also benefit hepatic steatosis.

Other Insulin Resistance-Associated Monogenic Conditions

Several monogenic conditions related to insulin resistance involve marked obesity (e.g., Alström and Bardet-Biedl syndromes), neurological diseases (e.g., myotonic dystrophy and Friedreich ataxia), or rapid aging (e.g., Werner syndrome).

Diagnostic and Predictive Molecular Testing in Monogenic Diabetes

Molecular testing for the primary causes of monogenic diabetes is widely available and should be considered for individuals with a moderate to high likelihood of a positive result. Testing is guided by clinical phenotype and the prevalence of mutations in the population.

Familial characteristics are also taken into account, as monogenic diabetes can coexist with type 1 or type 2 diabetes in families. Genetic testing is crucial for prognosis, treatment decisions, and screening family members. Where a genetic diagnosis is confirmed, phenotypically unaffected relatives should be tested to assess their future diabetes risk. Predictive testing should be accompanied by thorough counseling.

Care should be exercised, as monogenic diabetes can manifest in families with concurrent T1DM or T2DM. Therefore, the results of genetic testing must be interpreted alongside clinical findings. For instance, a patient diagnosed with glucokinase diabetes may also develop T1DM or T2DM.

In cases where a family member has a confirmed genetic diagnosis, asymptomatic relatives should undergo testing to assess their risk of future diabetes development. If the primary mutation phenotype involves diabetes, regular urine or blood testing may be preferable, as prospective testing offers limited additional benefit. Families seeking predictive testing should receive comprehensive counseling on potential implications.

Glucocorticoids

Glucocorticoids, named for their ability to elevate blood glucose levels, have the most significant impact on glycemic control among commonly prescribed medications. In the 1930s, it was observed that diabetic symptoms improved after either adrenalectomy or hypophysectomy, highlighting the crucial role of glucocorticoids in glucose homeostasis. This understanding was soon integrated into clinical practice, particularly after Hench et al.'s 1949 discovery of the potent anti-inflammatory effects of glucocorticoids.

The therapeutic application of glucocorticoids has increased significantly. According to the General Practice Research Database, nearly 1%

of the UK population uses oral glucocorticoids at any given time, with the prevalence rising to 2.5% among those aged 70 to 79 years. Inhaled corticosteroids are even more commonly used, with over 6% of the UK population utilizing them.

Glucocorticoids can worsen hyperglycemia in diabetic patients and significantly raise blood glucose and insulin levels in normoglycemic individuals when administered in high doses (equivalent to 30 mg/day or more of prednisolone). Long-term glucocorticoid therapy has been associated with impaired glucose tolerance or diabetes mellitus in 14–28% of patients. Those with a naturally low insulin response, particularly to glucose loading, are especially susceptible and may have a higher likelihood of developing type 2 diabetes (T2DM) later.

Glucocorticoids reduce insulin sensitivity in hepatic and peripheral tissues through post-receptor mechanisms. For instance, dexamethasone in adipocytes inhibits the expression of insulin receptor substrate 1 (IRS-1), a crucial protein in insulin signaling, which contributes to insulin resistance. However, this detrimental effect on insulin sensitivity may be partially mitigated by a glucose-independent stimulation of insulin secretion.

All glucocorticoids cause dose-dependent insulin resistance at doses exceeding 7.5 mg/day of prednisolone. The duration of glucocorticoid exposure does not seem to significantly affect this outcome, and hyperglycemia generally reverses upon discontinuation of the drug.

While oral glucocorticoids are most commonly associated with these issues, topically applied glucocorticoids can also cause severe hyperglycemia, particularly when used in high doses over large areas of damaged skin and under occlusive dressings. This risk is greater in children due to their higher body surface area to weight ratio. Although inhaled corticosteroids typically do not induce significant hyperglycemia, there has been a reported case of a patient with type 2 diabetes experiencing worsening glycemic control when prescribed high-dose fluticasone propionate. The hyperglycemic effects of glucocorticoids do not correlate with their anti-inflammatory or immunosuppressive potency. For instance, deflazacort, which has similar immunomodulatory effects as other glucocorticoids, causes less hyperglycemia than prednisone or dexamethasone.

Other frequently observed side effects of glucocorticoids include hypertension and sodium and water retention. Thiazide diuretics are not recommended to manage these side effects, as their hyperglycemic action can compound the effects of glucocorticoids.

Corticotropin (adrenocorticotropic hormone [ACTH]) or tetracosactide, previously used as alternatives to glucocorticoid therapy (such as in the treatment of multiple sclerosis exacerbations), are no longer recommended for therapeutic use.

Estrogen Replacement Therapy in Women with Diabetes

Hyperglycemia induced by hormonal contraceptives generally reverses upon discontinuation of the contraceptive pill. Current low-dose contraceptives do not seem to increase the risk of developing type 2 diabetes (T2DM) later, although high-dose pills used in the past may have posed such a risk.

Observational studies suggest that hormone replacement therapy (HRT) in women with T2DM is associated with a reduced risk of cardiovascular disease, which contrasts with findings in the general population where HRT does not reduce cardiovascular disease incidence in postmenopausal women. HRT formulations vary in estrogen type and dosage, progestogen type, and administration route, which likely influence cardiovascular risk and benefit in specific patient subgroups, such as those with diabetes. A placebo-controlled randomized study of 25 postmenopausal women with T2DM indicated that conjugated equine estrogen therapy (0.625 mg/day) improved blood glucose and lipid profiles. Another study involving 28 postmenopausal women with T2DM using continuous oral 17β-estradiol (1 mg) and norethisterone (0.5 mg) reported similar benefits.

The Women's Health Initiative study, which included over 160,000 postmenopausal women aged 50–79, found that those randomized to HRT had a lower incidence of self-reported diabetes compared to those given a placebo. This was true for both women taking conjugated equine estrogen alone and those taking it in combination with medroxyprogesterone acetate. These findings, along with a meta-analysis assessing HRT's effects on components of the metabolic syndrome in postmenopausal women, provide reassurance that estrogen replacement therapy can be considered for patients with diabetes.

Antihypertensive and Cardiovascular Agents

Thiazide Diuretics

The exact mechanism by which thiazide diuretics impair glucose tolerance is not fully understood. It was previously believed that both reduced glucose-stimulated insulin release and insulin resistance were responsible. However, recent evidence suggests that the impairment is due solely to reduced pancreatic insulin release, not decreased insulin sensitivity. The severity of glucose intolerance is strongly linked to the degree of hypokalemia. Potassium depletion inhibits the cleavage of proinsulin to insulin, leading to impaired insulin secretion, which is reversible upon restoring normal potassium levels. This results in postprandial hyperglycemia, with elevated proinsulin levels between meals potentially downregulating insulin receptors in peripheral tissues. This effect is observed in both non-diabetic individuals and those with type 2 diabetes, but not in type 1 diabetes patients who receive exogenous insulin.

β-Adrenoceptor Antagonists

β-Adrenoceptor antagonists affect glucose homeostasis at multiple points. Long-term studies indicate that these agents induce insulin resistance, possibly due in part to weight gain. This diabetogenic effect is exacerbated when combined with high-dose thiazides. A recent meta-analysis involving 94,492 hypertensive patients found that β-adrenoceptor antagonists were associated with a 22% increased risk of new-onset diabetes, with a higher risk in patients who had higher baseline body mass indexes and fasting glucose concentrations.

Calcium-Channel Blockers

Calcium-channel blockers have been shown in both in vitro and in vivo studies to impair glucose metabolism, although clinically significant hyperglycemia is rare and typically associated with excessive dosages. Verapamil, for example, inhibits the second phase of glucose-stimulated insulin release by blocking calcium uptake into the cytosol of β-cells. It also inhibits sulfonylurea and glucagon-induced insulin secretion. Hyperglycemia and metabolic acidosis are well-documented in cases of verapamil poisoning, with animal studies suggesting that the hyperglycemia results from a combination of impaired insulin release, insulin resistance, decreased insulin-mediated glucose clearance, and increased action of circulating catecholamines. Serum glucose concentrations have been found to correlate directly with the severity of calcium-channel blocker poisoning.

Other Drugs

β-Cell Toxins

Some drugs act as direct β-cell toxins, potentially causing permanent, often insulin-dependent diabetes. A notable example is streptozotocin, a nitrosourea compound used experimentally to induce insulin-dependent diabetes in rodents and as chemotherapy for inoperable or metastatic insulinoma in humans.

Pentamidine, which treats Pneumocystis infections in AIDS patients, is similar to another diabetogenic agent, alloxan. Pentamidine can destroy β-cells, initially causing insulin release and transient hypoglycemia, followed by diabetes. This effect is most pronounced when pentamidine is administered intravenously, but it can also occur through aerosol inhalation.

In a study involving 128 AIDS patients treated with pentamidine for Pneumocystis infections, nearly 40% experienced significant glucose homeostasis abnormalities. Specifically, 5% developed hypoglycemia, 15% experienced hypoglycemia followed by diabetes, and 18% developed diabetes alone. Risk factors for these glucose abnormalities included higher doses of pentamidine, elevated plasma creatinine concentrations, and severe anoxia.

Studies on Drug Effects on Adipocytes

Recent studies show that certain drugs have direct impacts on adipocytes, leading to insulin resistance, which hampers glucose uptake and inhibits lipolysis. Additionally, these drugs can impair the differentiation process from pre-adipocytes to mature fat cells.

β2-Adrenoceptor Agonists

β2-Adrenoceptor agonists stimulate insulin secretion; however, this is counteracted by increased hepatic glucose output, resulting in net hyperglycemia. High doses of β2-agonists, such as salbutamol, ritodrine, and terbutaline, are frequently used to treat asthma and premature labor, often causing hyperglycemia. In some cases, diabetic ketoacidosis has been reported in previously non-diabetic pregnant women. Continuous nebulization of β2-agonists for severe asthma can also lead to hyperglycemia. These effects are most pronounced in patients with type 1 diabetes mellitus (T1DM). When combined with dexamethasone, as in preterm labor treatment, the resulting hyperglycemia can be severe, even in normoglycemic patients. Consequently, the National Institute for Health and Clinical Excellence (NICE) advises using alternatives to β2-adrenoceptor agonists in diabetic women requiring tocolysis to avoid hyperglycemia and ketoacidosis. Other agents like epinephrine, dopamine, and theophylline can also induce hyperglycemia through similar mechanisms.

Diazoxide

Diazoxide, a non-diuretic benzothiadiazine derivative with potent vasodilatory effects, was previously used for hypertensive crises but is now rarely indicated for this purpose. It remains useful in cases of inoperable insulinoma and to treat severe hypoglycemia following sulfonylurea overdose. The typical dosage for insulinoma treatment ranges from 100 to 600 mg/day, administered in divided doses.

Diazoxide acts on the β-cell membrane to open the ATP-dependent potassium channel, hyperpolarizing the membrane and inhibiting insulin secretion, which can cause hyperglycemia after just a few doses.

Somatostatin Analogs

Somatostatin inhibits insulin secretion and also suppresses counter-regulatory hormones like growth hormone and glucagon. In individuals without diabetes, this typically maintains euglycemia. Octreotide, a somatostatin analog used for neuroendocrine tumors, has varying metabolic effects in T1DM and type 2 diabetes mellitus (T2DM). In T1DM patients treated with exogenous insulin, the suppression of glucagon and growth hormone decreases hepatic glucose production, potentially lowering blood glucose levels and/or insulin requirements. In T2DM patients, the inhibition of endogenous insulin secretion may predominate, leading to hyperglycemia. There is evidence that octreotide treatment can result in hyperglycemia in these patients.

Somatostatin Analogs and Glucose Metabolism

Somatostatin analogs have complex effects on glucose metabolism, particularly in patients with conditions like acromegaly, where glucose homeostasis is already compromised. These analogs reduce insulin resistance caused by elevated growth hormone levels but also suppress insulin secretion from pancreatic β-cells. The overall impact on glucose metabolism depends on the balance between these two effects, which can sometimes lead to worsened glucose control even as growth hormone concentrations improve.

Octreotide, leveraging its ability to suppress insulin release, has proven effective in managing refractory hypoglycemia resulting from acute sulfonylurea poisoning or quinine treatment.

Anti Rejection Drugs and Diabetes Risk

Post-transplantation diabetes mellitus (PTDM) has been reported in non-diabetic adult transplant recipients receiving ciclosporin (cyclosporine). Animal studies suggest that cyclosporine may cause reversible damage to pancreatic β-cells, contributing to the development of PTDM.

Immunosuppressive Drugs and Diabetes Risk

Pancreas allograft biopsies from transplant patients treated with cyclosporin demonstrate histological changes indicative of islet cell damage, including cytoplasmic swelling, vacuolization, and apoptosis. Studies indicate that the incidence of post-transplantation diabetes mellitus (PTDM) rises progressively over time, particularly with newer cyclosporine formulations that achieve higher blood concentrations due to improved gastrointestinal absorption. This higher cumulative exposure to ciclosporin correlates with an increased risk of diabetes.

Similarly, up to 28% of adults receiving tacrolimus (FK506), a potent immunosuppressive agent, develop PTDM. Recent trials suggest that using low-dose tacrolimus (0.15–0.2 mg/kg/day) may mitigate this risk. Altered insulin and glucagon responses to arginine in patients treated with these drugs indicate a dysfunction in the β-cell–α-cell axis within the pancreatic islets. Fortunately, reducing the dosage of both cyclosporine and tacrolimus can often reverse their diabetogenic effects.

Recent advancements in immunosuppressive protocols, aimed at minimizing steroid and nephrotoxic drug use, have led to increased use of non-nephrotoxic agents like mycophenolate mofetil and sirolimus. The association of these agents with PTDM remains uncertain, with conflicting study results on sirolimus suggesting both increased and non-increased risks of PTDM.

α-Interferon Therapy

α-Interferon therapy has been linked to the development of both type 1 and type 2 diabetes mellitus, occasionally with ketoacidosis. Autoimmune mechanisms are suspected to play a role in these cases.

Psychiatric Disorder Medications

Antipsychotic Agents

While hyperglycemia occasionally occurs with conventional antipsychotic drugs, newer atypical antipsychotics like clozapine and olanzapine are frequently associated with the onset of new diabetes mellitus and exacerbation of pre-existing diabetes. The causal relationship between antipsychotics and diabetes remains under scrutiny due to the presence of traditional diabetes risk factors in many affected patients.

Before the advent of antipsychotics, rates of diabetes in individuals with severe mental illness were already high.

Potential mechanisms linking antipsychotics to diabetes include hepatic dysregulation via antagonism of hepatic serotonergic mechanisms. Weight gain, often associated with fasting hyperglycemia and hyperinsulinemia, suggests insulin resistance as a contributing factor. Some in vitro studies also indicate a possible direct effect of antipsychotics on insulin secretion. In some cases, blood glucose levels may normalize upon discontinuation of the medication.

Antipsychotic Agents

The use of atypical antipsychotics is associated with an increased risk of glucose intolerance and diabetes mellitus. Estimates of the attributable risk of diabetes linked to atypical antipsychotics vary, ranging from 0.05% for risperidone to 2.03% for clozapine. Despite this risk, the absolute excess risk attributed to these medications is generally considered low, implying that most individuals prescribed antipsychotics will not develop diabetes. Nonetheless, baseline screening and regular monitoring are recommended to promptly identify and manage any adverse metabolic effects associated with treatment.

Antidepressants

Depression is prevalent among individuals with diabetes, and certain antidepressant medications can impact plasma glucose and insulin levels. For instance, the tricyclic antidepressant nortriptyline has been shown to worsen glycemic control and reduce insulin concentrations in animal studies. Additionally, there is a documented case of clomipramine causing symptomatic hyperglycemia that resolved upon discontinuation of the drug but recurred upon rechallenge. Selective serotonin reuptake inhibitors (SSRIs) such as fluoxetine and fluvoxamine induce hyperglycemia in animal models by enhancing serotonergic neurotransmission, which increases catecholamine release from the adrenal medulla while suppressing insulin secretion. However, these effects do not appear to be clinically significant in humans. In fact, SSRIs and other antidepressants have demonstrated benefits in improving glycemic control, potentially by reducing appetite, alleviating depression, and enhancing compliance with antidiabetic treatments.

Other Drugs

Asparaginase (), used in the treatment of acute lymphoblastic leukemia, predictably impairs glucose tolerance due to insulin resistance. In clinical trials involving children, asparaginase administration resulted in hyperglycemia in 10% of cases, all of which exhibited glycosuria.

Synthetic steroid derivatives with androgenic properties, such as oxymetholone and danazol, are known to impair glucose tolerance likely by inducing insulin resistance at a post-receptor site. Increased glucagon secretion may also contribute to their diabetogenic effects.

Nicotinic acid, prescribed for dyslipidemia treatment, can occasionally induce severe hyperglycemia. However, adverse effects of this nature were not observed in clinical studies evaluating its efficacy and safety.

Each of these medications requires careful consideration of potential metabolic effects when prescribed to patients, particularly those with existing metabolic disorders like diabetes. Regular monitoring and prompt intervention are essential in managing any adverse effects that may arise.

Gatifloxacin and Other Drug-Induced Hyperglycemia

Gatifloxacin, a fluoroquinolone antibiotic, has been associated with an estimated incidence of hyperglycemia around 1%. Reported cases include both new-onset diabetes and exacerbation of existing diabetes mellitus in affected patients. The precise mechanism underlying gatifloxacin-induced hyperglycemia remains unclear; however, animal studies suggest potential inhibition of insulin secretion or increased secretion of epinephrine as contributing factors.

Transient hyperglycemia has also been observed following treatment or overdose of various commonly prescribed medications, including non-steroidal anti-inflammatory drugs (NSAIDs), isoniazid, nalidixic acid, carbamazepine, encainide, benzodiazepines, and mianserin. These instances are documented primarily through anecdotal reports.

Treatment of Drug-Induced Hyperglycemia

The management of clinically significant drug-induced hyperglycemia varies depending on the causative agent:

- Glucocorticoid-Induced Hyperglycemia: High doses of glucocorticoids commonly lead to hyperglycemia. If this occurs during thiazide treatment, reconsideration of the need for the drug is recommended. If a diuretic is necessary, substituting with a lower dose of furosemide or bumetanide may be considered. Alternatively, adjusting the dosage of bendroflumethiazide to a lower level (e.g., 2.5 mg/day) or switching to another class of antihypertensive medication may be appropriate.

- Steroid-Induced Diabetes: In cases where withdrawal of glucocorticoid therapy is not feasible, managing hyperglycemia with "steroid-sparing" immunosuppressive drugs, such as methotrexate or mycophenolate mofetil, could be considered. These drugs are intended to reduce the required dosage of glucocorticoids, potentially minimizing the risk of developing steroid-induced diabetes mellitus.

These strategies underscore the importance of vigilant monitoring and individualized management of drug-induced hyperglycemia to mitigate adverse metabolic effects in affected patients.

CHAPTER THIRTEEN
ENDOCRINE DISORDERS CAUSING DIABETES

Key Points

Endocrine causes of diabetes primarily result from an excess of hormones that counteract insulin secretion or action:
- Glucagonomas and somatostatinomas, rare islet cell tumors, produce hormones that inhibit insulin secretion and action.
- Thyrotoxicosis commonly causes mild glucose intolerance but rarely progresses to diabetes.
- Acromegaly, almost always due to growth hormone-secreting adenomas, disrupts glucose homeostasis in up to 50% of cases.
- Other endocrinopathies like primary aldosteronism and hyperparathyroidism can also disturb glucose homeostasis.

Introduction

This chapter focuses on endocrine disorders that lead to hyperglycemia, where treating the underlying endocrinopathy can normalize blood glucose levels. These conditions are primarily characterized by excessive secretion of "counter-regulatory" hormones that oppose insulin action, either by inhibiting its secretion or its effectiveness.

Acromegaly

Acromegaly results from excessive growth hormone (GH) secretion, predominantly due to pituitary adenomas larger than 1 cm in diameter (macroadenomas). It affects approximately 60 individuals per million and is caused by GH-secreting adenomas in 99% of cases. Rarely, it can also arise from excess GH-releasing hormone (GHRH) or other conditions like multiple endocrine neoplasia type 1 (MEN1). The condition is often present for many years before diagnosis, allowing time for characteristic physical changes to develop.

Features of Glucose Intolerance in Acromegaly

Glucose intolerance or diabetes is prevalent in acromegaly due to the direct hyperglycemic effects of excess GH. Overt diabetes is reported in 19–56% of patients, with impaired glucose tolerance affecting 16–46% . Higher levels of GH correlate with increased diabetes incidence. Insulin resistance, induced by GH, impairs insulin action in the liver and peripheral tissues. This resistance exacerbates when GH stimulates lipolysis, increasing non-esterified fatty acids that further hinder glucose utilization. Initially, pancreatic compensation may maintain euglycemia, but over time, beta-cell compensation diminishes, leading to hyperglycemia.

Cushing Syndrome

Cushing syndrome results from excessive glucocorticoid levels, either exogenously from therapeutic use or endogenously due to ACTH-secreting pituitary adenomas, adrenal tumors, or ectopic ACTH secretion. It leads to characteristic physical changes and metabolic disturbances, including diabetes, hypertension, and cardiovascular complications.

Management of Cushing Syndrome

Successful management of Cushing syndrome includes surgical resection of tumors or radiotherapy, supplemented with medical options like ketoconazole or metyrapone for symptomatic relief. Post-treatment, patients may necessitate lifelong hydrocortisone replacement due to adrenal insufficiency. While glucose intolerance often improves following treatment, persistent obesity and metabolic issues may persist.

Pheochromocytomas: Causes and Symptoms

Pheochromocytomas, arising from adrenal chromaffin cells, secrete catecholamines causing symptoms such as headaches, sweating, and tachycardia, with hypertension observed in 80-90% of cases. These tumors can be hereditary or sporadic, often diagnosed via molecular genetic testing. Hyperglycemia associated with pheochromocytoma results from catecholamines inhibiting insulin secretion and promoting hepatic glucose production through adrenergic receptor stimulation

Case Presentation: Emergency Management of Pheochromocytoma

A patient presented urgently with severe chest pain and hypertension (blood pressure 240/130 mmHg). On admission, blood glucose was 27 mmol/L. Increased urinary catecholamine excretion indicated a right adrenal pheochromocytoma, confirmed by (a) computed tomography, (b) scanning with 131I-metaiodobenzylguanidine, and (c) positron emission tomography with 18F-fluorodeoxyglucose. Laparoscopic tumor removal resulted in resolution of both diabetes and hypertension.

Diagnosis and Management of Pheochromocytoma

Pheochromocytomas are diagnosed by detecting elevated levels of catecholamines through 24-hour urine collections measuring epinephrine, norepinephrine, and their metabolites. acid measurement is inadequate due to its high false-negative rate. In cases requiring more sensitivity, serum normetanephrine and metanephrine measurements are recommended. Imaging via MRI or CT aids in tumor localization. Treatment involves surgical adrenalectomy, often performed laparoscopically unless malignancy is suspected. Preoperative preparation involves meticulous alpha-receptor blockade followed by beta-blockade to prevent hypertensive crises during manipulation and cardiovascular collapse post-removal. Adrenolytic drugs like mitotane may be used in malignant cascs.

Outcome of Pheochromocytoma and Glucose Tolerance

Surgical removal of the tumor corrects metabolic abnormalities and resolves hypertension. Prompt diagnosis and treatment are crucial for optimal patient outcomes.

Mechanisms of Hyperglycemia in Pheochromocytoma

Hyperglycemia in pheochromocytoma results from catecholamines inhibiting insulin secretion and promoting hepatic glucose production through adrenergic receptor stimulation..

Other Endocrine Conditions Affecting Glucose Tolerance

Glucagonoma

Glucagonoma, a rare tumor of the pancreatic alpha cells, manifests with symptoms such as necrolytic migratory erythema and diabetes. Surgical removal is the primary treatment, though metastatic cases may require additional therapies.

Somatostatinoma

Somatostatinomas, arising from delta cells in the pancreas or duodenum, cause diabetes and steatorrhea. Diagnosis involves elevated fasting somatostatin levels and imaging with CT or MRI. Treatment includes surgical resection or palliative measures for metastatic disease.

VIPoma

VIPomas secrete VIP, leading to pancreatic cholera syndrome characterized by watery diarrhea, hypokalemia, and hypercalcemia. Surgical debulking is the mainstay of treatment.

CHAPTER FOURTEEN
PANCREATIC DISEASES AND DIABETES

Introduction

Pancreatic diseases can lead to diabetes, although they account for less than 0.5% of all diabetes cases. Several conditions affect the pancreas, damaging both exocrine and endocrine components, often impairing beta-cell function.

Acute Pancreatitis

Acute pancreatitis ranges from mild edema to severe necrosis, with symptoms such as sudden epigastric pain, nausea, and vomiting. Common causes include alcoholism and gallstones. Metabolic abnormalities like hyperglycemia and elevated lipase levels are typical, with imaging showing pancreatic edema. Transient hyperglycemia is common, resolving without insulin, but severe cases can lead to permanent diabetes.

Chronic Pancreatitis

Chronic pancreatitis involves irreversible exocrine tissue damage, often necessitating insulin due to glucose intolerance. Causes vary by region, with alcohol abuse predominant in the West and tropical pancreatitis more common in developing countries. Genetic factors like mutations in PRSS1 and SPINK1 can contribute.

Tropical Calcific Pancreatitis

A form of chronic pancreatitis prevalent in low-income countries, characterized by calcification of pancreatic ducts, leading to diabetes.

Hereditary Hemochromatosis

An inherited disorder causing iron deposition in pancreatic islets, leading to diabetes secondary to islet cell damage.

Table 15:1   Islet Cell Changes in Chronic Pancreatitis

This table summarizes the changes observed in different cell types within islets in chronic pancreatitis.

Cell Type	Observed Changes
Beta Cells	Reduced number and mass due to cell death. Impaired insulin secretion.
Alpha Cells	Relative increase in number compared to beta cells. Disruption in glucagon secretion patterns.
Delta Cells	Altered somatostatin production.
PP Cells	Changes in pancreatic

	polypeptide secretion.
Islet Structure	Fibrosis and atrophy of islet architecture. Inflammatory infiltration.

Secondary Hemochromatosis

Conditions like thalassemia major, necessitating frequent blood transfusions, often lead to substantial iron overload and subsequent pancreatic damage, frequently resulting in diabetes. The duration of illness and the number of transfusions are closely correlated with the severity of glucose intolerance. It has been hypothesized that iron overload might trigger autoimmune attacks on the β-cells, contributing to diabetes development.

Pancreatic Neoplasia

Pancreatic adenocarcinoma ranks as the fifth leading cause of cancer-related deaths and its incidence is on the rise. Prognosis remains poor with a less than 3% five-year survival rate. While diabetes has long been linked with pancreatic adenocarcinoma, the nature and strength of this association remain debated. A meta-analysis suggested a twofold increased risk of pancreatic cancer in individuals with diabetes exceeding 5 years. However, other studies argue that the cancer may precede and induce diabetes, supported by observations of diabetes improvement post-tumor resection. Conversely, some studies suggest diabetes may protect against pancreatic cancer. Tropical chronic pancreatitis is associated with a 100-fold higher risk of pancreatic carcinoma.

Pancreatic Surgery and Diabetes

Diabetes frequently complicates pancreatic resection for various indications. The incidence and severity of diabetes post-surgery correlate with the extent of distal segment resection, where islets are most abundant. One study indicated diabetes development in 56% of cases following distal resection. Subtotal pancreatectomy is more likely to result in diabetes compared to procedures like lateral pancreaticojejunostomy and pancreaticoduodenectomy (Whipple procedure). Total pancreatectomy invariably leads to diabetes. Managing diabetes following pancreatectomy is challenging, often characterized by wide blood glucose level fluctuations and heightened insulin sensitivity due to glucagon deficiency. Patients may benefit from frequent small meals and multiple small insulin doses, while some cases may benefit from subcutaneous insulin infusion pumps. Patients are ideal candidates for whole pancreas or islet cell transplantation. Associated exocrine pancreatic insufficiency should also be addressed, requiring low-fat, high-carbohydrate, and high-protein meals along with pancreatic enzyme therapy to manage steatorrhea and stabilize blood glucose.

Cystic Fibrosis

Cystic fibrosis is a multisystem disorder characterized by recurrent airway infections, pancreatic insufficiency, abnormal sweat gland function, and urogenital dysfunction. It is an autosomal recessive disorder caused by mutations in the CFTR gene. The most common mutation, deletion of phenylalanine at position 508 (ΔF508), leads to abnormally thick secretions, resulting in pancreatic ductular obstruction, dilation, and subsequent pancreatic insufficiency. Clinical manifestations include steatorrhea, failure to thrive, recurrent lung infections, hepato-biliary complications, and symptoms of fat-soluble vitamin deficiencies such as night blindness. While the disease affects 1 in 2500 live births in Caucasian populations, its prevalence is significantly lower in Africans and Asians.

Diabetes in Cystic Fibrosis

The incidence of diabetes in children with cystic fibrosis is 2-3%, approximately 20 times higher than in the general population. Incidence rises steadily through adolescence, with up to 25% of patients in their twenties developing diabetes and an additional 50% showing glucose intolerance. Damage to pancreatic β-cells secondary to exocrine pancreatic degeneration is the primary factor in diabetes pathogenesis. Additional mechanisms include enhanced glucose absorption and autoimmune attacks on β-cells. Interestingly, diabetes is more prevalent in patients homozygous for ΔF508 than in heterozygotes. Diabetes onset is insidious, characterized by a delayed, flattened, and prolonged insulin secretory response to glucose. Ketoacidosis is rare, though most patients require insulin therapy. Improved treatment of lung disease in cystic fibrosis has increased patient survival into adulthood, consequently raising diabetes prevalence. Chronic microvascular complications are increasingly common.

Management

While some patients may initially respond to sulfonylureas, most eventually require insulin therapy. Insulin not only controls diabetes but also improves body weight and pulmonary and pancreatic function. Regular screening for diabetes using oral glucose tolerance tests or serial HbA1c measurements should start in adolescence. Dietary management in patients with cystic fibrosis and diabetes mirrors that in chronic pancreatitis patients. A carbohydrate and protein-rich diet with fat restriction is recommended. Oral pancreatic enzyme therapy helps improve nutrient digestion and absorption, with enteric-coated lipase preparations controlling steatorrhea. However, higher strengths of lipase can predispose to fibrosing colonopathy.

Conclusions

While rare, secondary diabetes due to pancreatic disease holds significant clinical implications.

Proper treatment of the underlying pancreatic disease is crucial, and genetic disorders should be identified to screen family members. Diagnosis requires a high index of suspicion, with suggestive symptoms including features of pancreatic disease (steatorrhea, unexplained weight loss, or back pain) and severe diabetes in the absence of a family history of diabetes.

CHAPTER FIFTEEN
CLINICAL PRESENTATION OF DIABETES

Key Points

Patients with type 1 diabetes (T1DM) typically present with classical symptoms such as thirst, polydipsia, and polyuria. On the other hand, type 2 diabetes mellitus (T2DM) may present with complications, including diabetic ketoacidosis (DKA) or non-specific symptoms like tiredness and repeated infections.

Diabetes presents a diverse range of initial symptoms, often mimicking other conditions. The classic symptoms of T1DM, including acute onset thirst and weight loss, contrast with the often asymptomatic nature of T2DM. Early diagnosis through screening is crucial due to the potential for long-term complications, such as macrovascular (e.g., myocardial infarction, stroke) and microvascular diseases (e.g., neuropathy, retinopathy).

Clinical Considerations at Presentation

Understanding patient perspectives and beliefs about diabetes is essential during diagnostic consultations. The impact of diagnosis on individuals varies widely and can influence their long-term management and outlook. Differentiating between types of diabetes based on clinical history and initial symptoms guides immediate prognosis and therapeutic decisions.

Types of Diabetes

Diabetes classification remains debated, categorized broadly as T1DM (autoimmune destruction of β-cells), T2DM (insulin resistance or β-cell dysfunction), monogenic diabetes, and secondary forms like those due to pancreatic diseases or steroid-induced conditions. Each subtype requires tailored management strategies based on its underlying pathology.

Management Implications

The decision for insulin therapy hinges on clinical presentation, with clear indications such as DKA or significant weight loss with ketonuria and glycosuria. Early recognition and intervention can mitigate risks associated with diabetes-related complications, emphasizing the importance of personalized treatment plans.

Clinical Features of Diabetes Presentation

Thirst and Urinary Symptoms

Thirst, polydipsia, and polyuria are common in diabetes, with type 1 diabetes (T1DM) often presenting with acute symptoms. The choice of sugary drinks exacerbates symptoms. Nocturia is a clearer indicator in assessing urine frequency, crucial for diagnosis.

Renal Threshold and Glycosuria

Diabetes involves glucose escaping into urine when plasma glucose exceeds renal threshold. This threshold varies widely (6–14 mmol/L) among individuals and increases with age, affecting symptoms and clinical presentation.

Age-Related Considerations

With advancing age, the renal threshold and thirst perception change, impacting symptom recognition and dehydration risk. Chronic hyperglycemia alters vasopressin sensitivity, delaying thirst despite rising plasma osmolarity, especially problematic in older adults.

Weight Loss

Significant weight loss often signals diabetes onset, particularly in T1DM. However, its absence doesn't exclude the condition, as symptom onset may vary. In contrast, weight loss in type 2 diabetes (T2DM) can result from deliberate dietary changes or insulin deficiency affecting muscle and fat metabolism.

Infections

Undiagnosed diabetes may manifest through recurrent yeast infections or more severe sepsis cases. Candidiasis and skin infections are common, particularly in T1DM, highlighting the importance of early blood glucose control.

Blurred Vision

Sudden changes in plasma glucose levels can lead to blurred vision, typically following acute diabetes onset or hyperosmolar states. Educating patients on temporary visual changes due to glucose fluctuations is crucial to avoid unnecessary concerns and interventions.

Rare Infections

Diabetes increases susceptibility to severe infections like necrotizing fasciitis and mucormycosis, underscoring the need for vigilance in clinical assessment and management.

Diabetic Ketoacidosis (DKA)

Diabetic ketoacidosis (DKA) arises due to severe insulin deficiency, accompanied by elevated levels of counter-regulatory hormones. It is characterized by hyperglycemia, acidosis, and ketonuria, primarily affecting patients with T1DM, although it can also occur in some with T2DM. Symptoms of DKA include hyperglycemia (thirst, polyuria, polydipsia), malaise, muscle cramps, and severe abdominal pain with vomiting that mimics surgical emergencies. Recognizing these signs is critical to avoid administering anesthesia, which can be fatal if DKA is present. Clinical signs such as dehydration, Kussmaul respirations (deep, sighing respirations), and a sweet-smelling breath (acetone odor) are evident. Awareness that not all individuals can detect acetone odor underscores the need for multiple diagnostic tools. Severe cases may progress to coma, necessitating urgent blood glucose, urinary ketone, and arterial blood pH assessments for prompt treatment.

The absence or deficiency of insulin prevents glucose uptake into tissues (muscle, fat, liver), leading to dysregulated secretion of counter-regulatory hormones (glucagon, growth hormone, catecholamines). This dysregulation accelerates triglyceride breakdown into free fatty acids, increasing gluconeogenesis and subsequently elevating blood glucose levels. Beta-oxidation of free fatty acids produces ketone bodies (β-hydroxybutyrate, acetoacetate, acetone), with acetone imparting the characteristic breath odor. Metabolic acidosis results from ketone body release into circulation, depleting acid buffers.

Hyperosmolar Hyperglycemic Syndrome (HSS)

Hyperosmolar hyperglycemic syndrome (HSS) is exclusive to T2DM patients, characterized by profound dehydration often preceded by days of ill health. Typical symptoms include confusion, focal neurologic deficits mimicking stroke, and dehydration. Formerly known as hyperosmolar non-ketotic coma, HSS involves mild ketosis at diagnosis due to residual insulin secretion suppressing ketogenesis but insufficiently controlling hyperglycemia. Hyperosmolarity itself may further limit lipolysis and ketogenesis. HSS accounts for 10–30% of hyperglycemic emergencies and is increasingly seen in hospital admissions as T2DM prevalence rises, with up to two-thirds of cases previously undiagnosed.

Macrovascular Presentations

Acute Myocardial Infarction (AMI): Elevated blood glucose levels, seen in impaired glucose tolerance and diabetes, increase ischemic heart disease risk. Stress hyperglycemia during AMI worsens outcomes similarly to established diabetes, with mortality rates notably higher compared to normoglycemic individuals.

Acute Stroke: Hyperglycemia at stroke onset predicts poor functional recovery and increased mortality, highlighting the need for blood glucose control in acute stroke management. The impact of stress hyperglycemia in non-diabetic patients mirrors that in diabetic patients, with worse tissue function impairments.

Microvascular Presentations

Eye Presentations: Symptomatic vision loss may herald T2DM diagnosis, with long-standing hyperglycemia causing silent tissue damage and potentially severe retinopathy. Retinal examinations are crucial for early detection and management of sight-threatening conditions.

Foot Lesions

Foot lesions may serve as initial signs of diabetes, with a notable lifetime risk of foot ulcer development in diabetic individuals. Peripheral neuropathy contributes to sensory, motor, and autonomic dysfunction, leading to reduced pain sensation, dry skin, and callus formation. Detection of foot ulcers often coincides with concomitant peripheral arterial disease (PAD), significantly affecting healing rates and increasing major amputation and mortality risks.

Pregnancy

Gestational diabetes mellitus (GDM) pathogenesis is characterized by physiological insulin resistance during pregnancy. Exogenous insulin requirements in T1DM show minimal change until approximately 18 weeks' gestation, followed by a linear increase until around 28 weeks' gestation. Screening at 24–28 weeks' gestation is recommended due to heightened insulin resistance later in pregnancy, balancing sensitivity with intervention opportunities. After a pregnancy complicated by GDM, the risk of recurrence in subsequent pregnancies varies.

CHAPTER SIXTEEN
THE AIMS OF DIABETES CARE

Key Points

- People diagnosed with diabetes should not be viewed merely as passive recipients of healthcare but rather as individuals managing a condition with significant medical, personal, and social consequences.
- Optimal diabetes management involves active participation of the person with diabetes alongside a multidisciplinary healthcare team.
- Management should address acute hyperglycemic symptoms and life-threatening emergencies, while also focusing on long-term complication prevention through lifestyle and pharmacological interventions.

Introduction

Diabetes represents a chronic, incurable condition associated with heightened risks of premature mortality and cardiovascular diseases, as well as microvascular complications affecting kidneys, nerves, and eyes. Effective management hinges on improving glycemic control to mitigate microvascular complications, complemented by a comprehensive approach to cardiovascular risk factors to reduce associated morbidity and mortality.

Individuals living with diabetes bear the primary responsibility for managing their condition, dedicating a significant portion of their time to self-care compared to limited interactions with healthcare professionals. Thus, structured and purposeful consultations with diabetes healthcare teams, whether in clinical, telephonic, or educational settings, are crucial to maximize patient benefit.

St. Vincent's Declaration

The 1980s marked a pivotal shift in diabetes care philosophy from viewing patients as passive recipients to recognizing them as active partners in their treatment. This transformation culminated in the St. Vincent Declaration, where stakeholders emphasized patient responsibility and collaborative care with healthcare professionals to enhance diabetes management globally.

The Diabetes Care Team

Diabetes care is multidisciplinary, involving a spectrum of healthcare professionals dedicated to supporting individuals with diabetes. This team-oriented approach ensures personalized care and empowers patients to manage their condition effectively across primary and specialist care settings. Continuity of care is pivotal, ideally facilitated by consistent healthcare providers or through meticulous record-keeping in settings with transient care providers.

Improving Consultation Outcomes

Given the limited time available during consultations, preparation by both patients and healthcare providers is essential for optimizing interaction efficiency and patient outcomes. Effective communication and shared decision-making further enhance the efficacy of healthcare visits, fostering a collaborative approach to managing diabetes.

Before Your Appointment

- Prepare two or three key questions you want to ask.
- Make a list of all medications, including vitamins and supplements.
- Note down details of your symptoms, when they started, and what makes them better or worse.
- Arrange for an interpreter or communication support if needed.

- For support, think about bringing a friend or relative.

During Your Appointment
- In the event that you are unclear, don't be afraid to ask for clarification. For example, say, "Can you repeat that? I still don't understand."
- Request explanations in writing if you are unfamiliar with any terms.
- Take notes or have someone accompany you to jot down important details.

Before Leaving Your Appointment

- Ensure you have covered everything on your list of questions.
- Confirm your understanding by summarizing what was discussed, for example, "Can I confirm I understood what you said?"

- Know the next steps in your treatment plan, including any follow-up appointments or tests.
- Ask about whom to contact if you have further questions or issues.
- Inquire about support groups or reliable information sources.
- Request copies of any letters or reports written about you.

After Your Appointment

- Document what was discussed and any next steps in your treatment plan.
- Schedule any recommended tests and mark the dates in your calendar.
- Follow up on test results if not received as expected, asking for them if necessary.
- Seek clarification on what the results mean for your condition.

Interactions Between Diabetes Patients and Healthcare Professionals

The consultation or educational program should foster a mutual understanding of diabetes between healthcare professionals and patients. Rather than a one-sided delivery of care, these interactions should empower individuals with diabetes to actively participate in decision-making and care planning. Encouraging questions and providing clear explanations, along with written documentation when needed, enhances patient engagement and improves outcomes. Regular reviews of management plans through collaborative dialogue between healthcare professionals and patients are crucial for building effective partnerships and maintaining effective care. Contact information should be readily available so individuals with diabetes know where to seek assistance for any ongoing concerns.

Following Diagnosis

The period following a diabetes diagnosis is critical for long-term management. Patients often require substantial support and education to navigate the complexities of diabetes care. Tailored medical examinations and personalized care plans, including treatment-oriented goals, are essential to accommodate individual needs and preferences.

Diabetes Education

Educational initiatives play a pivotal role in equipping individuals with diabetes with the knowledge and skills necessary for effective self-management. This ongoing process should be adapted to reflect current medical advancements and individual circumstances, encouraging behavioral changes essential for long-term health.

Table 17:1

	Glycated Hemoglobin (HbA1c) Lipid Profile	Blood Pressure (mmHg)Lipid Profile	Lipid Profile
ADA	< 53 mmol/mol (< 7.0%)	< 140/90	LDL < 100 mg/dL
			HDL > 40 mg/dL for men, > 50 mg/dL for women
			Triglycerides < 150 mg/dL
EASD	< 53 mmol/mol (< 7.0%)	< 130/80	LDL < 1.8 mmol/L (< 70 mg/dL)
			HDL >

			1.0 mmol/L (men), > 1.2 mmol/L (women)
			Triglycerides < 1.7 mmol/L (150 mg/dL)
IDF	< 48 mmol/mol (< 6.5%)	< 130/80	LDL < 2.5 mmol/L (< 95 mg/dL)
			HDL > 1.0 mmol/L (39 mg/dL)
			Triglycerides < 2.3 mmol/L

			(200 mg/dL)
NICE	< 48 mmol/mol (< 6.5%)	< 130/80	Total cholesterol < 4.0 mmol/L (< 155 mg/dL)
			LDL cholesterol < 2.0 mmol/L (77 mg/dL)

ADA: American Diabetes Association, EASD: European Association for the Study of Diabetes, IDF: International Diabetes Federation, NICE: National Institute for Health and Clinical Excellence.

The Diabetes Control and Complications Trial and the UK Prospective Diabetes Study (UKPDS) have firmly established that maintaining lower levels of glycemia significantly reduces the risk of long-term microvascular complications in both Type 1 and Type 2 diabetes. To mitigate these risks, authoritative bodies such as the American Diabetes Association (ADA), European Association for the Study of Diabetes (EASD), and governmental entities like the National Institute for Health and Clinical Excellence have established stringent glycemic targets for individuals with diabetes. Despite these recommendations, achieving optimal control remains challenging for many individuals with diabetes. Healthcare providers should actively explore barriers to achieving these targets with their patients and offer appropriate adjustments in treatment or additional education as necessary.

Hypoglycemia poses a significant obstacle to achieving optimal glycemic control and is one of the most uncomfortable, inconvenient, and feared side effects of diabetes medications. It is essential to discuss the frequency and severity of hypoglycemic episodes with patients and provide guidance on prevention strategies. For individuals treated with insulin, ensuring ready access to glucose sources such as glucose tablets, concentrated glucose solutions, and glucagon is critical. Caregivers and family members should also be trained in administering these treatments in case of severe hypoglycemia, ensuring they are up-to-date and proficient in their use.

In some cases, achieving strict glycemic control may necessitate accepting a slightly less stringent target to avoid disabling hypoglycemia. This decision should be made collaboratively with the patient, considering individual circumstances and potential risks beyond hypoglycemia. The broader clinical context and the risk of complications specific to the individual should also guide discussions on setting realistic glycemic goals.

While glycemic targets receive significant clinical emphasis, findings from trials such as the Action to Control Cardiovascular Risk in Diabetes (ACCORD), Action in Diabetes and Vascular Disease: Preterax and Diamicron MR Controlled Evaluation (ADVANCE), and Veterans Affairs Diabetes Trial (VA-DT) highlight a nuanced approach. These trials indicate that intensive glycemic control may not necessarily prolong life, and in some cases, may increase cardiovascular mortality, particularly in individuals with longer diabetes duration. These outcomes underscore the importance of personalized glycemic targets based on individual health profiles and risks.

GLOSSARY

Acromegaly: A hormonal disorder that results from excess growth hormone (GH) and can cause glucose intolerance.

Adipokines: Bioactive peptides produced by adipose tissue that influence metabolism, including insulin sensitivity.

Adipose Tissue Hypoxia: A condition where reduced blood flow in adipose tissue leads to inflammation and metabolic disturbances.

Bariatric Surgery: Surgical procedures performed on the stomach or intestines to induce weight loss, often used to treat obesity and related metabolic conditions.

Body Mass Index (BMI): A measure of body fat based on height and weight, used to classify overweight and obesity.

Cushing Syndrome: A disorder caused by high levels of cortisol, leading to symptoms such as weight gain and glucose intolerance.

Diabetic Ketoacidosis (DKA): A serious complication of diabetes characterized by high blood sugar, ketone production, and metabolic acidosis.

Endoplasmic Reticulum (ER) Stress: Cellular stress in the ER affecting protein folding and contributing to insulin resistance.

Fatty Acids: Components of fat involved in energy storage and metabolism, which can impact insulin sensitivity and glucose metabolism.

Free Fatty Acids (FFA): Fatty acids released into the bloodstream during lipolysis, influencing glucose metabolism and insulin sensitivity.

Genome-Wide Association Studies (GWA): Research studies that look for genetic variations across the genome to identify associations with diseases, including diabetes.

Gestational Diabetes Mellitus (GDM): A form of diabetes diagnosed during pregnancy that can affect the health of both mother and baby.

Glucokinase MODY: A type of maturity-onset diabetes of the young (MODY) caused by mutations in the glucokinase gene, affecting glucose metabolism.

Glucagonoma: A rare pancreatic tumor that secretes glucagon, leading to hyperglycemia and other metabolic disturbances.

Glycosuria: The excretion of glucose in the urine, typically a sign of high blood sugar levels.

Hemochromatosis: A genetic disorder causing excessive iron accumulation in the body, which can lead to diabetes and other organ damage.

HNF1A, HNF4A MODY: Types of MODY caused by mutations in the HNF1A and HNF4A genes, affecting insulin production and glucose metabolism.

Hormone-Sensitive Lipase: An enzyme that breaks down stored fats into free fatty acids, regulated by hormones including insulin.

Hyperglycemia: Elevated blood glucose levels, a primary feature of diabetes.

Hyperosmolar Hyperglycemic Syndrome (HSS): A complication of type 2 diabetes marked by extremely high blood glucose levels and dehydration, without significant ketoacidosis.

Insulin Resistance: A condition where cells in the body respond poorly to insulin, leading to elevated blood glucose levels.

Insulin Sensitivity: The effectiveness of insulin in promoting glucose uptake by cells, often decreased in diabetes.

JNK and IKKβ-NF-κB Pathways: Inflammatory signaling pathways in adipose tissue that contribute to insulin resistance and metabolic disturbances.

Lipid Metabolism: The process by which fats are synthesized and broken down in the body, influencing energy balance and glucose metabolism.

Lipoprotein Lipase (LPL): An enzyme critical for the breakdown of triglycerides in lipoproteins, influenced by insulin and glucose levels.

Maturity-Onset Diabetes of the Young (MODY): A group of monogenic diabetes forms characterized by early onset and autosomal dominant inheritance.

Metabolic Acidosis: A condition where the body produces excess acid or cannot remove acid effectively, often seen in diabetic ketoacidosis.

Mitochondrial Dysfunction: Impaired function of mitochondria, the cell's energy producers, contributing to metabolic diseases like diabetes.

Neonatal Diabetes: A form of diabetes diagnosed in the first six months of life, often caused by genetic mutations.

Obesity: Excessive body fat accumulation, a significant risk factor for type 2 diabetes and other metabolic disorders.

Pheochromocytoma: A rare tumor of the adrenal gland that can cause excessive hormone release and lead to hyperglycemia.

Somatostatinoma: A rare tumor that secretes somatostatin, leading to glucose intolerance and other symptoms.

Splanchnic Glucose Disposal: The uptake and metabolism of glucose by the liver and other organs in the abdominal cavity.

Triglycerides: A type of fat found in the blood used for energy storage, high levels of which can impact glucose metabolism.

Type 1 Diabetes Mellitus (T1DM): An autoimmune condition where the body attacks insulin-producing beta cells in the pancreas.

Type 2 Diabetes Mellitus (T2DM): A metabolic disorder characterized by insulin resistance and relative insulin deficiency, often associated with obesity.

Urinary Nitrogen Excretion: A measure of nitrogen in the urine, indicating protein breakdown, which is influenced by insulin levels.

VIPoma: A rare endocrine tumor that secretes vasoactive intestinal peptide, affecting glucose metabolism and other bodily functions.

Visceral Fat: Fat stored within the abdominal cavity around internal organs, more strongly associated with insulin resistance and metabolic risk than subcutaneous fat.

Waist Circumference: A measure of abdominal obesity, which is a better predictor of metabolic risk than BMI alone.

Dear Reader,

Thank you for choosing to read 'Comprehensive Diabetes Care'. Your support means a lot to me as an author dedicated to providing valuable content on diabetes diagnosis and care.

If you found this book informative and helpful, I would greatly appreciate it if you could take a moment to leave an honest review on Amazon. Your feedback not only helps me improve as a writer but also assists other readers in making informed decisions about their reading choices.

Please feel free to share your thoughts on what you liked or how the book has benefited you. Your reviews are incredibly valuable and contribute to the book's success.

Thank you once again for your support and for being a part of this journey with me.

Warm regards,
Dr. Barry R. Putney.

www.ingramcontent.com/pod-product-compliance
Lightning Source LLC
Chambersburg PA
CBHW071914210526
45479CB00002B/412